The
LOST ART
of
DYING

The
LOST ART
of
DYING

REVIVING FORGOTTEN WISDOM

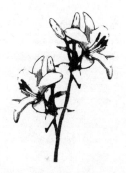

L. S. DUGDALE

Artwork by Michael W. Dugger

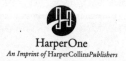

HarperOne
An Imprint of HarperCollinsPublishers

HarperOne

The pieces of art in the gallery are by Michael W. Dugger, who holds exclusive rights to these works. They are used here by permission and cannot be reproduced or copied outside of this context without further permission from the artist at mwdugger.com.

The content of this book has been carefully researched by the author and is intended to be a source of information and guidance only. Although the reflections and suggestions contained herein can benefit the general public, readers are urged to consult with their physicians or other professional advisers to address specific medical or other issues that may arise. The author and the publisher assume no responsibility for any injuries suffered or damages or losses incurred during or as a result of the use or application of the information contained herein.

Names and identifying characteristics of some individuals have been changed to preserve their privacy.

FIRST EDITION

Designed by Terry McGrath

Library of Congress Cataloging-in-Publication Data

Names: Dugdale, Lydia S., 1977– author.
Title: The lost art of dying : reviving forgotten wisdom / L.S. Dugdale ; artwork by Michael W. Dugger.
Description: First edition. | New York, NY : HarperOne, 2020 | Includes bibliographical references.
Identifiers: LCCN 2019031054 (print) | LCCN 2019031055 (ebook) | ISBN 9780062932631 (hardcover) | ISBN 9780062932662 | ISBN 9780062979759 | ISBN 9780062932655 (ebook)
Subjects: LCSH: Death. | Terminal care. | Loss (Psychology)
Classification: LCC BD444 .D84 2019 (print) | LCC BD444 (ebook) | DDC 155.9/37—dc23
LC record available at https://lccn.loc.gov/2019031054
LC ebook record available at https://lccn.loc.gov/2019031055

---

20 21 22 23 24 LSC 10 9 8 7 6 5 4 3 2 1

For my patients
and
In memory of my grandmother
Ella May Newkirk Ulrich
April 22, 1921–March 29, 2019

CONTENTS

The
LOST ART
of
DYING

CHAPTER ONE

DEATH

I regret that we resuscitated Mr. W. J. Turner. He was a little
old man, aged further by the cancer that had invaded his
bones and lungs and brain. He had eluded death for so long
that his daughters had begun to whisper of his immortality.
They believed, or so they told themselves, that he might live
forever.

When his organs began to shut down like falling dom-
inos, he was admitted to the oncology ward at my hospital.
His daughters assured the medical team that he would "beat
this cancer." They told the nurses, "Do everything you can to
keep him alive." The night Mr. Turner died, none of us knew
for certain whether his family understood the immensity of

1

his disease or the misery that would doubtless accompany his prognosis.

I had never met Mr. Turner. In fact, in that uncanny set of circumstances only experienced by doctors and emergency medical technicians, I encountered his dead body before I met him. Human corpse before human being. Death before life.

I was talking with a patient in our emergency room when the code alarm sounded. A college student with asthma was attempting to explain the impetus for her hospital visit in two-word increments. She had—*wheeze*—been at a—*wheeze*—party and her friends—*wheeze*—were . . .

"Code Blue, Nine West! Code Blue, Nine West!" An authoritative voice from the hospital's overhead speaker system interrupted the wheezing. These broadcasts always sounded the same, the voice steady and deep, unfazed by the fact of death.

"That's me. Have to run. Back later," I blurted, racing to the elevator. It was faster to take the elevator than the stairs to any code above the fourth floor—especially in the middle of the night. As the elevator doors parted, a fellow member of the code team, Amit, greeted me. "Wonder if we know the patient," he said. "Man, codes on the cancer floor are always bad."

He was right. The cancer ward rarely felt hopeful—at least to us doctors. The patients were desperately sick, often having failed chemotherapy or radiation. It felt like an eternal winter—full of bulbs that never blossom.

Medical professionals are partly culpable for engineering

such circumstances. We have mastered the art of offering third- and fourth-line chemotherapies for ostensibly untreatable cancers. We tell ourselves that we want to give hope, but a last-ditch effort at chemotherapy is rarely the hope our dying patients need. By focusing on fixes, we ignore finitude. And we accompany our patients to their deaths in the hospital with chemotherapy coursing through their veins.

I sighed when I reached Mr. Turner's emaciated body lying cruciform on the hospital bed. This wouldn't go well. Why resuscitate? Everyone shared the thought, but no one said it. His pale brown skin was stretched tautly over a skeletal frame. The lifeblood drained, his body was cool to the touch.

We quickly established hierarchy, the reigning principle of the teaching hospital. The senior, or "attending," physician bears moral and legal responsibility for a patient's care and oversees the team of students and doctors at various levels of training. The attending physician is followed—in decreasing order of seniority—by the fellow, the senior resident, and the junior resident or intern. Then come the students from across the health professions. Nurses, therapists, chaplains, and social workers round out the crew. This team approach guarantees multiple levels of oversight and ensures that someone who knows the patient will nearly always be in the hospital.

The intern that night knew Mr. Turner best and began to tell his story while those of us assigned to the task of resuscitation began our work. "Eighty-eight-year-old man, history of metastatic prostate cancer, status post–radical prostatectomy, chemo, and radiation, readmitted two weeks ago with worsening mental status and bone pain, found to have new brain and bone mets." Without flinching, he delivered this medicalized eulogy for a medicalized death.

The head of our code team asked me to insert the central line—a large catheter—into a main blood vessel in the groin. Through this line we would push medications to stimulate the heart. Two other doctors were attempting to introduce a breathing tube into Mr. Turner's airway. One doctor kneeled over the body as he compressed cancer-laden ribs. Another prepared to shock the heart electrically. Nurses worked at placing an intravenous line in the arm and dispensing medications that sometimes help to revive the dead.

We labored efficiently and with precision. We had perfected the knowledge and technique for resuscitating dead bodies. Although the odds were against us, it worked. "I've got a pulse," Amit said.

We all paused. The pulse did not waver, and the nurse manager took charge. "Okay. Let's get his bed cleaned up and get this man to the ICU." Mr. Turner was a man again, a human *being*, no longer a human corpse. *Being*, the present participle of *be*, implies existence. He was alive. We had forced life into his lifeless body.

Patients whose cardiopulmonary resuscitation (CPR) is successful are always transferred to intensive care. This is because the very act of *pulmonary* resuscitation requires the insertion of a breathing tube into the patient's airway. This tube then attaches to a mechanical ventilator that breathes for the patient until the lungs prove their independence. Ventilators require the around-the-clock staffing and monitoring of the intensive-care unit (ICU).

Resuscitation complete, Amit and I tore off our paper gowns and latex-free gloves. We wiped the sweat from our foreheads. Our bodies had assumed various contorted postures during the twenty or so minutes we had worked to resuscitate Mr. Turner, and now we straightened our crooked frames.

"Can't believe we got him back."

"I'll call the family," I said.

And that was it. Having checked "revive the dead" off our to-do list, we dispersed to other duties.

I waited in the ICU until Mr. Turner's daughters arrived. Even though I wasn't his primary physician, I wanted to talk with them. I doubted that they had been told that he was dying and that his cancer was consuming him. They needed to know. There was no question that his heart would stop again, probably soon, and I hated to think of repeating what had just occurred. All the life support in the world couldn't ultimately save him.

His family appeared promptly—hair and clothing so well assembled that one would hardly guess they had been sleeping just minutes before.

We sat together in the "fishbowl," a glass-walled conference room close to Mr. Turner's bed. I explained what had happened. They thanked us for saving his life. I reiterated, gently, that there was no doubt that his cancer was killing him and that his heart would not likely hold out under the stress of the disease. I asked whether they would consider going without cardiac resuscitation, were his heart to stop again.

The eldest daughter did not flinch. "No, Doctor," she replied. "We are Christians, and we believe that Jesus can heal. We believe in miracles. You do whatever you can to keep him alive."

This has always struck me as something of a paradox. It seems curious that the people who believe most fervently in divine healing also cling most doggedly to the technology of mortals.

Aggressive Measures

But Mr. Turner's daughters aren't the only religious people who choose aggressive measures. The sentiment is, in fact, quite common among the devout. A recent Harvard study found that patients with high levels of support from their religious communities are more likely to choose aggressive life support and to die in intensive-care units. They were also less likely to enroll in hospice. Why might this be?

The researchers had many suggestions. Perhaps religious communities are ill-informed when it comes to medicalized death, which makes it difficult to know when a person is actually dying. Or, since so many religious people believe that God cures through doctors, limiting life support might seem obstructive to divine healing. Still other religious groups place a high value on the "sanctity of life," possibly raising ethical concerns about actions that appear to curtail the number of days a person could live.

Recognizing that such patients might receive guidance from religious leaders on medical care at the end of life, the researchers decided to ask clergy what they understood about care of sick and dying people. Interestingly, they discovered that clergy knew little about palliative and other care at the end of life. They had little insight into potential harms and overestimated the potential benefits of invasive procedures. The researchers concluded that pastoral zeal to encourage faith in God might inadvertently enable congregants to choose unhelpful treatments associated with greater suffering.

Perhaps some of these factors contributed to the Turner daughters' dogged insistence on resuscitating their dying father.

Raising the Dead—Again

"Code Blue, Five South, Intensive Care. Code Blue, Five South, Intensive Care." The same somber voice bellowed from the speaker system on high. About ninety minutes had passed since we had resuscitated Mr. Turner, and I was in the doctors' workroom writing up admission orders for my asthmatic college student. "Guess who coded this time," Amit said as we ran toward Mr. Turner's body. It was not a question.

For the second time that night, we encountered the body of a deceased Mr. Turner. Again we rhythmically compressed the cancerous ribs—the ribs we had unintentionally fractured not two hours earlier. Again we pushed medicines into the intravenous lines hoping that they would animate his heart. And then, as if bestowed with some sort of power to raise the dead, we successfully brought Mr. Turner back to life. Again.

The Turner daughters thanked us. We each returned to our respective stations as though nothing had changed: they to the bedside of their beloved father, Amit and I to the workroom.

But something had changed. We had resuscitated a dead man not once, but *twice*, in the same night. And he wasn't just any man. He was an impossibly frail man drowning in the tempest of advanced illness. Amit beat me to it. "He's not going to survive the night."

"Bad Blood" and Burial Insurance

The Harvard study found that highly religious people, regardless of race or ethnicity, were more likely to die medicalized deaths. But when the researchers took race and ethnicity into account, they found that Hispanic and black patients, like Mr. Turner, had a disproportionately greater chance of receiving aggressive end-of-life care *and* were more likely to have high levels of support from their religious communities.

Black and Hispanic patients prefer more aggressive interventions at the end of life. In study after study, researchers have found this to be true. But no one is exactly sure why.

One theory is that the medical profession has betrayed the

trust of minority populations through years of egregious ex-
perimentation. Perhaps the most notorious American example is the "Tuskegee Study of Untreated Syphilis in the Negro
Male," also known as the Tuskegee Syphilis Study, conducted
by the US Public Health Service in conjunction with Alabama's historically black Tuskegee University between 1932
and 1972. The study aimed to observe the natural progression
of untreated syphilis in rural African American men.

Investigators enrolled about six hundred sharecroppers
from Macon County, Alabama. Of these, nearly two-thirds
had contracted syphilis before the study began; the remaining
one-third were healthy. There was no known cure for the disease at the time, and none of the infected men was even told
that he had syphilis—only "bad blood." In exchange for their
participation, the men were given free medical care, meals,
and burial insurance.

The culture of medical research and practice at this point
in history was distinctly paternalistic. Doctors made decisions
on behalf of their patients, and researchers made decisions on
behalf of their subjects. The doctor knew best. Although, by
definition, paternalism limits the ability of patients to make
autonomous health-related decisions, it was usually understood to be exercised in a spirit of protective goodwill. Doctors were paternalistic because they were paternal—good
parents making decisions for the good of their children.

Nothing about the Tuskegee experiments was paternalistic
in this sense; the Tuskegee study was purely exploitative. A
mere fifteen years after the study began, penicillin was estab-

lished as the cure for syphilis. Yet the researchers again failed to inform the men that they had syphilis or that they could be treated for it. And because syphilis is transmitted sexually and from mother to fetus, many partners and children suffered as a result. The study continued for another twenty-five years until a journalist exposed the abuses.

Tuskegee may be infamous, but it was not exceptional. US researchers experimented on prisoners, sex workers, and mentally impaired patients in the Guatemalan syphilis experiments of the 1940s; on American prisoners for Albert Kligman's dermatology experiments during the 1950s and 1960s; and on disabled children in the Willowbrook, New York, hepatitis experiments from the 1950s to the 1970s. The list goes on. It's no wonder that some patients, not excepting Mr. Turner and his family, regard with suspicion the seeming eagerness of physicians to withhold chest compressions or remove life support.

And Again . . .

Amit and I had barely resettled ourselves in the workroom when the voice announced, "Code Blue—" We didn't wait to hear the location. We ran, unfazed by death.

A code in the real world looks nothing like a code on television. The team is substantial. Doctors, nurses, respiratory therapists, chaplains, and social workers all have roles. Adrenaline charges through arteries, and—despite best efforts—blood spurts out of veins. Sometimes we can shock a rebellious heart into obedience for an easy fix. Sometimes resuscitation takes so long that the patient suffers brain damage. It nearly always appears chaotic to outside observers, but it's a carefully orchestrated pandemonium.

Resuscitations can be disturbing to watch, so we typically usher family members away from codes. By Mr. Turner's third death, however, there was nothing to hide. As for a woman in prolonged labor, modesty had been lost, and the nakedness of death lay in plain view of Mr. Turner's daughters.

This time our superhuman powers had faded. Mr. Turner's heart ignored our most ardent pleas. After twenty minutes of CPR, the code team leader performed the ritual that seals the fate of the recently deceased: he called off the code. This time, there would be no raising the dead.

Medical professionals know well that when the heart stops, the brain fails to receive the oxygen-rich blood it requires to thrive. After even a few minutes, brain tissue begins to die. By ten minutes, doctors expect irreversible brain damage.

The purpose of CPR, then, is to oxygenate the blood (via "mouth-to-mouth" or breathing tube) and to circulate it around the body by performing chest compressions. It's critical to get the blood to the brain quickly, which is why Amit and I ran to the patient when the code alarm sounded. But artificially oxygenating the blood remains inferior to the body's natural capabilities. If resuscitation attempts continue for fifteen or twenty minutes and CPR is unsuccessful, the medical team worries about the possibility of brain damage. After twenty to thirty minutes, we usually surrender our efforts and call off the code.

When we ceased compressing Mr. Turner's chest, we declared him dead—another medical ritual. The declaration of death typically involves shining a penlight into the eyes to check for pupil constriction. Mr. Turner's pupils did not flinch. Amit then placed his stethoscope on Mr. Turner's chest, and, while he listened, we observed whether the stethoscope rose and fell with his breathing. No movement. No sound. Total stillness.

No matter how much a bed is needed, the nurses in our hospital always provide the family a couple of hours with the body to grieve. Then the corpse is transferred to a gurney and delivered headfirst to the morgue. Only the living ride the gurney feetfirst.

We offered our condolences to the Turner daughters, answered their questions, and left them with the chaplain and social worker. We then set off to complete the paperwork of death.

Conveyor Belts and Processing Plants

Mr. Turner died his three deaths while I was still a resident physician, but his skeletal form has haunted me ever since. In our hospital, CPR is a daily occurrence. We routinely compress disintegrating ribs, raise the dead, and prevent their resting in peace through mechanical ventilation. But we almost never resuscitate the same body three times in the same night.

Somehow, the way Mr. Turner died felt like a personal and professional failure. Despite giving him the best medicine has to offer, we had contributed to his dying poorly. Yes, he died the way his daughters wanted, or thought they wanted. But it was as awful to inflict as it was to witness. In short, Mr. Turner's story illustrates the ways that we—as individuals and as a society—fail to die well.

The physician and writer Victoria Sweet has in recent years been calling for the practice of slow medicine. Sweet argues that just as slow food is healthier than fast food, slow medicine is healthier than fast medicine.

Aristotle would doubtless have approved. The ancient Greek philosopher extolled the virtue of practical wisdom—that practice of careful deliberation that helps us see the good of a whole. A thoughtful, deliberative approach to medicine is good for patients. It minimizes the risks and burdens of treatment. It prevents doctors from burning out and quitting. Slow medicine requires practical wisdom.

But health-care systems aren't structured for slow medicine. One doctor describes hospitals as "conveyor belts and processing plants," invoking the so-called *dis*assembly lines of the early twentieth-century slaughterhouses that inspired Henry Ford's automobile assembly lines.

Ford aimed at efficiency. "The idea is that a man must not be hurried in his work—he must have every second necessary but not a single unnecessary second," he wrote in his memoir. As the Model T progressed down the assembly line, interchangeable parts and subdivided labor led to increased output and decreased costs. Medicine, with its efficiency standards, operates on much the same principle. When patients enter the hospital doors, they take their place on a conveyor belt. They are attended to by the efficient "subdivided labor" of doctor, nurse, therapist, and technician: each measures some detail, adjusts some device, or monitors for quality control.

There is a difference, however. Neither the automobile nor the slaughterhouse animal is able to protest. But the patient can.

Early on in my medical career, I wondered why patients didn't try to resist the forward sweep of the medical conveyor belt. Why didn't they protest that surgery or refuse that chemotherapy? But then I met patients who were overwhelmed by their experience of health care. Medical decisions require the mental fortitude to weigh the risks and benefits of treatment. My patients were sick, frightened, and frenzied. Medical decisions require in-depth knowledge of human anatomy as well as a familiarity with the medical vernacular. My patients lacked such expertise.

If health-care systems bewilder patients by their sheer complexity, doctors make things more perplexing. We might tell patients, "There's always a chance that the back pain will improve with surgery," or, "There's always a chance that the cancer will shrink with another round of chemotherapy." We humans are wired to survive; we want to take the chance for life.

And so most patients stay on the belt as passive recipients of medical technique and knowledge. They remain *patients* in the truest sense of the word: a patient as one who is acted upon, the recipient of the doctor's agency.

But what's so bad about patients being conveyed from the hospital door through treatments and back out the door again? Isn't that simply the efficiency that characterizes a successful medical experience?

The problem is that this conveyor belt does not stop as death approaches. Yet this is precisely the point at which we most need slow medicine and the exercise of practical wisdom.

The belt moves just as swiftly and efficiently for the relatively healthy young man with an abnormal heart rhythm as for the frail elderly man who suffers from the same. In both cases, the cardiologist suggests an implantable heart device, the proven technology to prevent death from a potentially fatal heart rhythm. It's true that the device fixes the problem, but is it appropriate for a frail older man who is already suffering from late-stage dementia? Would the surgery to implant the device cause more discomfort and disorientation than the possibility of dying from a painless arrhythmia? Is life extension always the goal of health care?

When patients and their families are educated or encouraged to ask such questions, discussions become fruitful. Most doctors are more than happy to discuss the wisdom of various procedures or interventions. But if no one speaks up, if no one presses pause, the medical machine keeps moving. And the elderly patient goes to the operating room to receive his implantable heart device.

It's not wrong for doctors to apply the knowledge we possess to cure a patient. We are simply following standards that have been delineated by researchers. But is it wise to act as if death is avoidable and thereby attempt to delay death indefinitely? In failing to guide patients to die wisely, doctors fail at the professional commitment "to do no harm." Where is the wisdom on dying wisely?

I grew up in a household where talk of death was common. My grandfather Norman Ulrich had been a B-17 bomber pilot in World War II. In flight school, his airplane malfunctioned during takeoff and crashed, beheading his flight instructor. Grandpa broke his pelvis and back and was hospitalized for several months. He turned down an honorable discharge in favor of returning to flight school, which was granted.

During the war, he was shot down over a potato field in Germany and taken prisoner. In prison camp, he concocted creative recipes using stale bread crusts to keep his fellow prisoners and himself from starving. In early 1945, he survived one of the coldest winters on record by huddling during breaks in forced marches around a hand-built cookstove. Even after he and his fellow prisoners were liberated by General Patton in April of 1945, death was never far from his mind.

Some of my earliest memories are of Grandpa's frankness about his mortality. He secured burial plots for my grandmother and himself while he was still a young healthy man. He was on great terms with the undertaker. He had planned the order of service years before his funeral. And when his grandchildren started talking of tattoos, he threatened to write us out of his will—a document he had worked out many decades prior to his death. For more than twenty years, my siblings and I flew back to Chicago for important events and holidays just in case it would be Grandpa's last. He died at age ninety-five.

Medical practice has provided me with ample opportunity to emulate my grandfather—to reflect on mortality and what it takes to die well. Yet medicine's solution for the problem of dying poorly remains elusive. How might we—the current and future patients that we are—die wisely? I pondered this question for years.

One day as I scoured journal articles for a writing project, I came across a clue. It is neither high-tech nor cutting-edge. In fact, the solution for the problem of medicalized dying dates back about six hundred years to medieval Europe. It is the *ars moriendi*, Latin for "art of dying," a body of literature that described practices for dying well. But to tell the story of the birth, life, and death of the *ars moriendi* requires now, as it did then, a musing on death itself.

Plague and Putridity

In the 1340s, an old disease struck Europe with renewed vigor—the bubonic plague. It was called "bubonic" after the Greek *boubōn*, meaning "groin," because infected individuals developed large lymph nodes, or "buboes," in the armpits and groin. It was also known as the Black Death, because the tips of the toes, fingers, and nose became necrotic and black from either gangrene or the collapse of the body's blood-clotting system. The first symptoms of illness preceded death by about a week. The plague was highly contagious and uniformly fatal for those who contracted it. It was caused by the tiny bacterium *Yersinia pestis* and required nothing more than a bite by an infected flea, a minuscule annoyance with deadly power.

Such fleas live on rodents, usually brown rats, which they in turn infect. Since fleas live short lives, new fleas feed on infected brown rats and themselves become infected. In the Middle Ages, this cycle would repeat itself—flea to rat, rat to flea. The rats carried the fleas westward from China to England. The fleas bit ankles as they went, infecting bodies from toe to head and infecting Europe from east to west.

Although the plague regarded no person as exempt, some of the wealthy did manage to escape—often to private villas outside urban centers that were free of infected rats. The Italian humanist Giovanni Boccaccio survived the plague's 1348 outbreak in Florence. He went on to publish *The Decameron* in 1353, documenting atrocities wrought by the plague. He writes specifically about Florence, but his stories typify experiences across Europe.

According to Boccaccio, the plague completely unraveled the fabric of Florentine society. Despite the city's best efforts to keep out the sick, practice good sanitation, and petition the Almighty for divine protection, the rats and fleas invaded. The Florentines quickly realized that doctors had nothing to offer. Medicine was powerless, and the advice of doctors useless. The plague spread easily, even with minimal contact. Boccaccio reports watching pigs tear through the rags of a plague victim.

They began "writhing about as if they had been poisoned," he says, and they died soon thereafter.

The only order that emerged from the chaos was the self-sorting by Florentines into three groups. Some holed themselves up as hermits inside their homes, permitting no one to enter or exit. They ate and drank modestly, fearful of inviting divine retribution for any reason. Others, recognizing that death was imminent, indulged their most hedonistic desires. They frequented taverns and the well-stocked private homes of residents who had fled or died of the plague. As Florence descended into total lawlessness, most houses became common property, their goods consumed by these pleasure seekers. The third group took a middle road, neither locking themselves up nor indulging their passions. They went out for strolls carrying flowers or sweet-smelling herbs, which they held up to their noses "to fortify the brain . . . against the stinking air that seemed to be saturated with the stench of dead bodies and disease and medicine."

Everywhere the people of Florence looked, they saw death. In order to save themselves, family members abandoned their sick. Parents deserted children, wives left husbands. If servants remained to care for dying masters, they sacrificed their lives in the effort. In Boccaccio's own words, "The number of people dying both day and night was so great that it astonished those who merely heard tell of it, let alone those who actually witnessed it." Historians estimate that as much as two-thirds of Europe's population died in this outbreak.

Boccaccio describes preplague Florentine customs with regard to care of the dying. Neighbor women would gather at the bedside, together with the family, to comfort and mourn. Once the sick had died, the women joined the kin in public displays of grief. The men filled a different role, waiting with the priests outside the house to transport the corpse to the church of the deceased's choosing.

These practices, together with all that was normal and familiar, disintegrated with the plague. No one gathered at the deathbed. No one waited outside the home to shoulder the coffin in a funeral march. And almost no clergy came when summoned. Instead, the poor seized the opportunity to make fast money by hiring themselves out to wealthy families to dispose of corpses. These corpse carriers did not worry too much about delivering bodies to preferred burial grounds. Rather, they deposited them in the nearest uninhabited graves.

The lower and middle classes proved an especially pathetic sight for Boccaccio. With no country villa to escape to and no servant's help at hand, they had little choice but to stay in their neighborhoods and die. Thousands fell ill each day and night. They died in their homes and in the streets. As Boccaccio put it, "The stench of their decaying bodies announced their deaths to their neighbors well before anything else did. And what with these, plus the others who were dying all over the place, the city was overwhelmed with corpses." Putrid bodies piled high. No living being could escape the spectacle and smell of death.

Who can fathom this scene? Although I have witnessed more people die than I can count, images of this intensity evade me. But it was in response to this unimaginable horror that the *ars moriendi* was born.

In its first iteration, the *ars moriendi* referred to a handbook on the preparation for death. Related books, including an illustrated version, began to develop throughout the 1400s—a time when premature death from plague, war, or famine was almost inevitable. A central premise was that in order to die well, you had to live well. Part of living well meant anticipating and preparing for death within the context of your community over the course of a lifetime.

Over centuries, the original *ars moriendi* grew into a sizeable literary genre. It shaped practices related to living and dying in the West for more than five hundred years, succumbing only to the arrival of an early twentieth-century society fixated on ushering in a modern age. Cultural habits began to change dramatically. The automobile promised independence. The suffragists brought liberation. Talking movies, television, and jazz music supplanted earlier modes of entertainment. Antibiotics and anesthesia offered life beyond life. Not only did we stop thinking about how to die well; our very culture became inhospitable to the art of dying.

A New *Ars Moriendi*

This book seeks to explain and to revive the *ars moriendi*—not in its original form, but in a manner that matches modern sensibilities. Although the art-of-dying literature was birthed within the context of the Western church, this is not a religious book. It *is*, however, a book on the wisdom of dying well derived from centuries of Western Judeo-Christian cultural practices. And for that reason, it does not avoid the influence of Judaism or of Christianity on habits of dying in the West. Nor does it ignore other existential dimensions.

This book accepts as a given that, when it comes to dying and death, we need to look backward in order to move forward. The arc of the book thus proceeds from the problem of medicalized and institutionalized dying through to a description of a revitalized *ars moriendi*.

In each chapter, I will consider an aspect of what it takes to die well and challenge you to reconsider your views of dying and death. I have already set up the problem in this first chapter by telling the story of Mr. Turner's three deaths. We do not die well, and conveyor-belt medicine will continue to carry us to bad deaths unless we hit "pause" in the system. Changing the way we die takes work.

What sort of work? I'll show you that dying well requires the recovery of a sense of finitude (Chapter Two) and the embrace of community (Three)—both central features of the original *ars moriendi*. But there's more. To die well we must guard against the excessive allure of the hospital as the destination for dying (Four) and recognize that our fears of death cannot be medicalized away but must be courageously confronted (Five). I'll explain the importance of regarding our own ailing bodies and accompanying others in their frailty (Six). Since living so as to die well requires deliberate reflection, we'll also consider possible roles for spirituality (Seven) and ritual (Eight). In the last chapter, I'll attempt to spell out for you a modern *ars moriendi*—a practical guide to living and dying well.

If the whole project sounds morbid to you, rest assured that it's not. The art of dying well starts with the art of living well. That's what we'll discuss in the pages that follow—how to live well with a view to the endgame.

CHAPTER TWO

FINITUDE

Each year Gertrude Capella comes to my office for her annual checkup. With age, Ms. Capella has lost neither memory nor feistiness. She has, however, lost most of her hearing. Practically deaf, Gertrude talks so loudly that the entire office hears her before they see her. On a recent visit, Ms. Capella spoke louder than ever.

I sat squarely facing her in the examination room, making sure she could read my lips. For the fifth time, I inquired whether she would consider purchasing hearing aids.

"Look, I'm ninety-four," she said. "If I wanted hearing aids, I should've bought them years ago. Now I won't get my money's worth."

She had a point. She was acknowledging her finitude and making decisions based on it.

Later I asked Ms. Capella about her views on cardiac resuscitation and life support—a requirement for Medicare's annual visit. She shocked me with her answer.

"You keep me alive at all costs, you hear me?" (I heard her.)

Although she seemed to understand that years of smoking had irreversibly damaged her heart and lungs, she wanted us to resuscitate her if her heart stopped. And despite her advanced lung disease and dependence on nasal oxygen, she insisted on a breathing tube and mechanical ventilation if needed. Ms. Capella would be content with nothing less than maximum life support.

My mind raced through the scenario that would inevitably play itself out. It made no sense to think of trying to resuscitate a heart that had long since exceeded its warranty. We might be able to restart it, but, like a car without gasoline, it would quickly sputter out again.

If CPR were only a matter of restarting the engine, it might not be so bad. But cardiac resuscitation requires manual rib compressions. And compressing the brittle ribs of an elderly woman with osteoporosis feels the same as breaking sticks in half for a summer evening bonfire—only without the good memories. If Ms. Capella's heart stopped and we tried to restart it, she would end up with multiple painful rib fractures.

If we were successful with the heart, she would find herself breathing through a mechanical ventilator. Given her terrible lung disease, she might never be able to live independently of a breathing machine. To top it off, she would likely die in the hospital. There would be no art to this sort of dying.

But she declined to discuss it. In her mind, the question she faced was whether she should choose to live a few days longer, and she had decided. And despite any scenario I might paint, she could not accept herself as finite and would do whatever she could to prevent that finitude from taking hold for good. She could not imagine her own death, except abstractly, in its relationship to money spent on hearing aids.

Our human life span is exceedingly short when juxtaposed with the existence of the universe. We are finite creatures in finite bodies. Yet, paradoxically, we cannot seem to fathom our own mortality. At least not in our current circumstances. Can we die well if we refuse to acknowledge our finitude?

People who want to die well must be willing to confront their finitude. We do not have to accept death, invite it, or wish for it. But we must be prepared to say, "Yes, I am human and therefore mortal. One day I will die." We cannot both cling to the indefinite extension of life and effectively prepare for death.

Hominem Te Memento

It used to be the case that human beings had much more contact with the dead. More women died in childbirth, more infants died before their first birthday, and more children died before adulthood. Those who survived childhood were expected to live until what we now think of as middle age.

Although global data gathering is a relatively new practice, the numbers from the past half century alone underscore this point. Worldwide average life expectancy increased from 52.5 years in 1960 to 72.2 years in 2017. In the United States, the average hovers around 79 years. In 1960, 12.2 percent of babies worldwide died before the age of one; by 2017, that number had fallen to 2.9 percent. Before the rise of the modern hospital (see Chapter Four), the care of the dying, including dying infants, occurred within the context of the home and community, where death could be seen, heard, touched, and smelled. People were more likely to have been able to imagine their own deaths, because they witnessed death regularly.

In contrast, our society today leaves little room for the contemplation of human finitude. To stave off thoughts of mortality, we like to keep everything around us looking new. We design our clothes to be fashionable for a year or two. Our technology is governed by the theory of planned obsolescence. Our built environment comes with the expectation that certain buildings be demolished and rebuilt every specified number of years. And more than ever, scientists and beauty experts alike are striving to find that elixir for infinite youth. Apart from our life-insurance policies, little reminds us of our mortality.

Even in the hospital, we no longer grow old or die—or at least we try to avoid discussing it. Most doctors feel ill-equipped to tell patients that they are dying. During my seven years of medical training I had only two workshops on the topic "how to deliver bad news," despite the fact that medical practice is replete with bad news. Our sixty-minute sessions hardly scratched the surface. Rather than focusing on specifics, such as "how to tell a patient she's dying of cancer," we focused on approach—setting the stage for a difficult conversation, inviting the patient or family to explain their understanding of the situation, and practicing empathy. There is no question that these techniques are important, but they fail to prepare young doctors for the high-stakes conversations they will inevitably have with their patients. And the better we are at staving off death with technology, the less likely we will cultivate such skills.

Some people do plan ahead and attempt to contemplate their own finitude, but it is still difficult to picture ourselves dead. We can visualize all sorts of other things that we have never experienced: what it might be like to ride in a hot air balloon, for example, or to vacation in Bora-Bora. We can watch videos and discuss such experiences. Yet somehow, no matter how much we read about death and no matter how many times Granddad repeats his story about seeing white light and hearing his name called when his heart stopped during surgery, we cannot imagine ourselves as nonexistent. We cannot grasp what it means. And this makes consideration of finitude even more challenging.

My patient, Ms. Capella, is not alone in her reluctance to contemplate her finitude. On the one hand, I want to suggest that this deficit in imagination is a modern phenomenon, compounded by contemporary commitments to youth and beauty and longevity. On the other hand, the ability to ignore our finitude is perhaps intrinsic to the experience of being human. Perhaps, depending on circumstance, we have always needed reminders of our mortality.

In the ancient world, victorious Roman generals paraded triumphantly through the streets before adoring crowds. Accounts of these "triumphs" vary, but typically the general was accompanied in his chariot by a servant whose one task was to whisper repeatedly in the general's ear, *Hominem te memento!* or, "Remember that you are but human!" The servant's role was to ensure that the general did not start thinking of himself as godlike, as immortal. Perhaps ordinary people—those who faced the burden of disease and hunger and manual labor—did not require such reminders. But those tempted to see themselves as immortal apparently did.

The question this prompts for us is this: Does comfortable modern Western life tempt us to see ourselves as immortal? If the answer is yes, which I suppose to be the case for many of us, we too need a reminder of our humanity. But what sort of prompts will suffice?

Memento Mori

The need for a constant reminder of mortality was not limited to triumphant Roman generals. The ancient Greeks thought about death as a matter of routine. Socrates taught that the principal goal of philosophers is to rehearse for dying and death. The ancient Hebrews agreed. Qohelet, the "Teacher" of Hebrew scripture, instructs his listeners to remember their God while they are young, "before the days of trouble come, and the years draw near when you will say, 'I have no pleasure in them'... and the dust returns to the earth as it was, and the breath returns to God who gave it." Prepare now, the Teacher says, for to dust you will return.

Such reminders of mortality from antiquity were forerunners to a visual reminder of death called memento mori. The term *memento mori* combines the Latin *memini*, "to remember, to bear in mind," with *morior*, literally, "to die." Taken together, the phrase serves as a warning: "Remember! You will die!" We have adopted the term in English today to mean a reminder of death.

Versions of the memento mori became popular in medieval Europe. They took many forms: painting, sculpture, music, literature, dance, jewelry, or relics such as skulls and locks of hair. Skeletons symbolized death, and winged skeletons suggested for some the possibility of life after death. Timepieces or hourglasses in paintings and on gravestones reminded viewers that life is fleeting. On the face of it, the idea of a memento mori might strike us as morbid. But in medieval Europe it was considered a vital tool for orienting life's priorities. Life was lived with a view toward death.

One genre of art related to the memento mori is the "vanitas painting," so named for another of Qohelet's famous reminders, "Vanity of vanities! All is vanity." Compared with the infinite, the logic goes, all that is finite is trivial, meaningless, futile. "Remember," the Teacher says, "you are dust, and to dust you shall return."

Vanitas paintings are still-life paintings meant to point to human finitude. For instance, in Philippe de Champaigne's 1671 painting titled *Vanitas*, three objects occupy a simple gray slab, which may be a shelf or tabletop—or the lid of a sarcophagus. The objects are set against a black backdrop. The first is a red tulip with yellow tips, its stem drawing continuously from the water that fills the bottom of the glass bud vase. It is still and still alive, but not for long—an appropriate object for a still life. The middle object, a skull, is still but no longer alive. The third is an hourglass; its sand is running—not still and not alive.

On the one hand, these objects signal that the shift from life (the tulip) to death (the skull) is only a matter of time (the hourglass). On the other hand, they might suggest that life, beauty, and time are fleeting and only death is certain. Regardless of Champaigne's intent, the simplicity of the composition makes it difficult for us to escape its significance as it hangs on the wall. *Remember that you will die!* I have often wondered whether patients such as Ms. Capella would approach the end of their lives differently if they had spent the last ninety years with a painting of a skull hung on the living-room wall.

Although the various types of memento mori were highly popular, they may have been too popular. They were so commonplace that many people stopped paying any attention to them. As in Boccaccio's Florence, the prospect of death barely affected some, sobered others, and made dedicated epicures of the rest. Something more was needed. In order to constrain the cultivation of hedonists and reinforce the need to prepare well for death, all forms of the medieval memento mori prompted the learning of the *ars moriendi*, or art of dying.

Scientia Mortis

The rancid rotting flesh that resulted from the mid-fourteenth-century plague made the memento mori seem like mere child's play. Who required a reminder of mortality when the stench of death was everywhere? Those Europeans who had survived the plague needed something much more concrete. They needed to know how to prepare for death and what to do when the Grim Reaper came knocking.

But there was a problem. Europe's leading social authority at the time, the Catholic Church, suffered from its own internal disease. From 1378 to 1417, two and later three men simultaneously claimed the papacy, splitting the church. Weakened by decades of internal political turmoil, this social authority had little nourishment to offer its hungry, plague-stricken flock.

The Council of Constance was convened and met from 1414 to 1418 to resolve the papal problem and address concerns of the neglected laity. At the top of the list? How to prepare well for death. One council member, the chancellor of the University of Paris, Jean Charlier Gerson, championed efforts to address this concern.

Gerson wrote prolifically. Among his works was a handbook that included a section entitled *Scientia mortis*, or "Knowledge of Death," which addressed the care of the dying. Little did Gerson know that the *Scientia mortis* would serve as a model for the *ars moriendi* literary genre that would transform how Europeans—and later Americans—approached death.

Gerson's work was not elitist; *Scientia mortis* aimed to instruct all members of the community—children and adults, clergy and laity—in the care of the dying. The work explained in concrete terms how to encourage the sick and dying, engage them in dialogue, and pray on their behalf. Gerson's handbook was meant for real-time use at the bedside of a dying friend—a "how-to" guide on the subject of dying well. It became popular, despite having, as one scholar put it, "the cut-and-dried, unleisurely manner of the service books."

Like any instruction manual, this *ars moriendi* source made for a dull read. But it would go on to prompt a rich literary art form.

Ars Moriendi

In 1415, an anonymous author published the *Tractatus artis bene moriendi*, or "Treatise on the Art of Dying Well," which was inspired by Gerson. Its title is considered the source for the Latin name of the genre—the *ars moriendi*.

Although more than six hundred years have passed, I have been repeatedly struck by the need for a similar handbook today. That's why I wrote this book. Although some of the original *ars moriendi* content is less relevant to the diverse and global twenty-first century, it nevertheless offers rich wisdom on how we might die well. What follows are some of its highlights.

First, we have to acknowledge the possibility of death while we are still healthy. The *ars moriendi* ignored the question of whether death is good or bad. Instead, it simply suggested that "to die well is to die gladly and willfully." Although we need not insist that the only people who die well are those who accept death and "die gladly and willfully," the *ars moriendi* hit the mark with its assertion that in order to die well, you must take mortality into account, even when death seems a long way off. Plenty of people die well even though they do not want to die. You can push back against death and still die well. But you cannot ignore death.

The *ars moriendi* also drove home the point that we die best in community. Rare is the person who dies alone and dies well. In fact, we might go so far as to say that it is *impossible* to die well if you die alone. Having said this, some of us might recall a relative who waited until everyone left the hospital room in order to die. Such a scenario is, in fact, quite common. People who tend to avoid burdening others throughout their lives also tend to allow themselves to die once everyone has gone to bed for the night. However, this sort of politeness should not be mistaken for dying alone. People who walk toward their mortality without moral support die poorly. I'll explore this more in the next chapter.

To mitigate the possibility of the lonely death, the *ars moriendi* provided specific instruction to community members. Family and friends were to gather at the bedside and broach the uncomfortable subject of death; no one was allowed to offer false hope about recovery from illness. Community members were to encourage the dying to repent of sin. In fact, so the logic went, it was better for the dying to fear for their physical well-being and turn to God than to believe that they are healed and ignore their souls. Community members were exhorted to pray for and read religious texts to the dying. Even if you weren't particularly close to the person who was dying, the *ars moriendi* suggested, you had a role to play. Dying in the fifteenth century was truly a community affair.

Consumers of the *ars moriendi* texts were most drawn to descriptions of the emotions the dying were expected to face. They learned that the dying might be tempted to fall into feelings of despair, disbelief, impatience, pride, and avarice, and the *ars moriendi* offered specific consolations for each of these temptations. Since it is hard to know, in advance, what dying really feels like, these descriptions helped people anticipate the complex set of feelings they might experience as they confronted their finitude.

Doing any task well requires effort, and dying is no exception. For this reason, the *ars moriendi* described concrete actions for the dying person to take, such as reciting short prayers and affirming beliefs through a series of questions and answers. These served as a sort of proxy for extreme situations, such as during plague outbreaks, when clergy were in short supply.

It is crucial in our modern pluralistic society to note that, despite its religious origins, the *ars moriendi* was under no delusion that its audiences would be particularly pious. The scholar Mary Catharine O'Connor notes that the author of the *ars moriendi* "makes it quite clear by repeated statements that the 'cunnynge of the crafte' of dying is not only for 'religious & devoute' men but also for 'carnall & seculer' men. As a matter of fact his inclusion of religious men sometimes sounds like an afterthought, as if he feared that his brethren might fall into the sin of complacence if he omitted them."

The *ars moriendi* was for everyone. It taught that *all* people—young and old, rich and poor, religious and not—should give attention to the art of dying well by living well throughout their lives. Building upon Gerson's handbook, the *ars moriendi* was intended to be "a complete and intelligible guide to the business of dying, a method to be learned while one is in good health and kept at one's fingers' ends for use in that all-important and inescapable hour." To make it an imperative: rehearse for death while you are healthy, and keep the instruction manual handy.

The instruction manual, or "complete and intelligible guide," was very much in vogue during the mid- to late fifteenth century. The elite were preoccupied with self-fashioning into "complete" ladies and gentlemen, and the printing press allowed for the wide circulation of self-help books on manners and social graces. Texts appeared on all categories of the finer arts: wielding table knives, engaging in conversation, chess, courtship, and even weeping. It is no wonder that a text on the art of dying would naturally find its way into this class of books.

Unlike guides on the art of conversation, however, the *ars moriendi* literature was not intended solely for the elite. Its distribution was facilitated by the return of Council of Constance members to their home countries in 1418 and bolstered by the introduction of the printing press shortly thereafter.

Several decades after the distribution of the first *ars moriendi* handbook, an abridged adaptation made the rounds. It was known simply as the *Ars moriendi* (with an uppercase *A*) and was composed primarily of illustrations made from woodcut prints. The author intended the illustrations to be interpretable without text, ensuring that all people, including the uneducated and illiterate, could prepare for death.

The Spread of the *Ars Moriendi*

We know that the illustrated *Ars moriendi* began circulating around 1450, but no one has identified the responsible artist. Many of the illustrations contain the monogram "E.S.," which we presume belonged to a German goldsmith and engraver who worked in printmaking at the time. Art historians customarily add the honorific "master" to describe an unidentified artist who achieved the level of master craftsman. There is no question that E.S. merits the title.

Master E.S.'s illustrated *Ars moriendi* focused on the most popular aspect of the *ars moriendi* textual version—the five temptations faced by the dying. Of his eleven woodcut prints, five depicted those temptations, and another five pictured their resolutions. This meant that the illustration of disbelief was paired with an image of encouragement in faith, despair was coupled with an illustration of comfort through hope, impatience with a print encouraging patience, pride with humility, and avarice with "letting go" of the earthly.

It is easy to imagine how constant suffering might tempt the dying to become exasperated and wish to "get it over with." Let's look more closely at the paired images that addressed the issue of impatience.

In the first illustration, a dying man lies in bed. He is angry. A bedsheet only partially obscures his naked body. He thrusts his left leg out from under the sheet to kick away an attendant, perhaps the doctor. A matronly woman stands in the background and makes excuses: "See how he suffers," she says, the words scrawled in Latin on the image. The bedside table is overturned. The floor is littered with a bowl, cup, knife, and spoon. A young woman stands at the foot of the bed, ready to serve a plate of food and drink, but she appears unsure of where to set them.

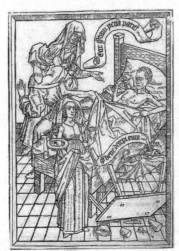

The Temptation of Impatience

Lest the observer think that such impatience is the

result of the illness itself, the illustrator has added a winged demon—an evil creature that lurks in the shadows of the dying man's bed and bears responsibility for this outburst. "How well I have deceived him!" he exclaims. Dying is not easy, the picture teaches, and we will be tempted to grow impatient.

This illustration is not pretty. In fact, it is easy to see how it might have provoked fear in the dying, had it not been paired with an image that brought relief. The accompanying illustration shows an angel who has come to the aid of the dying man, encouraging him to exercise patience. God the Father and Christ with his crown of thorns stand at the bedside—a display of loving solidarity with the suffering man.

Also at the deathbed stand four martyrs—*martyr* in Greek means "witness." These saints bear witness to the suffering of the dying man and are themselves living testimonies of misery redeemed. Stephen, who was stoned to death

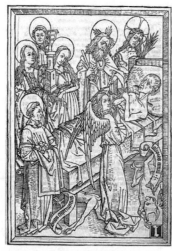

Comfort by Patience

in the first century, stands at the foot of the bed, with those same stones gathered in his arms. The third-century martyr Laurence, in the background, holds the gridiron on which he was burned to death, while his contemporary, Barbara, holds a model of a tower. Legend has it that Barbara's father locked her in a tower to keep her away from the seductions of the world. When she told her father that she had converted to Christianity, he beheaded her himself. Catherine, a fourth-century martyr, holds the wheel on which she was tortured. In studying these pictures, viewers would understand that the witnesses offer testimonies to the transcendent peace that enables the dying man to endure his present physical suffering.

The meaning of these medieval woodcut prints would have been perfectly intelligible to any fifteenth-century commoner. The question was how to obtain access to the prints. Although xylography, or the art of making woodcuts, had been practiced since at least the ninth century, western Europe required access to a steady supply of inexpensive paper in order for the illustrated *Ars moriendi* to become commercially viable. Finally, one hundred years after the bubonic plague, Europe's paper mills were in full production and woodcut prints emerged in their full glory. When Master E.S.'s illustrated *Ars moriendi* became widely available, the genre's popularity soared.

As they circulated more and more widely, the *ars moriendi* works were translated into many languages. In 1651, the Anglican cleric Jeremy Taylor published a decisively Protestant version called *The Rules and Exercises of Holy Dying*, and others followed. Eventually, the genre made its way to the United States and by the mid-nineteenth century was no longer especially religious; it had infiltrated mainstream culture. Advice on dying well appeared in health manuals, ballads, and poetry.

In her book on the American Civil War, *This Republic of*

Suffering, the historian Drew Gilpin Faust describes the secularization of the art of dying. She notes:

> By the 1860s many elements of the Good Death had been to a considerable degree separated from their explicitly theological roots and had become as much a part of respectable middle-class behavior and expectation in North and South as they were the product or emblem of any particular religious affiliation. Assumptions about the way to die remained central within both Catholic and Protestant faiths, but they had spread beyond formal religion to become a part of more general systems of belief held across the nation about life's meaning and life's appropriate end.

Dying well had become a universal concern. Now all people—religious and irreligious, old and young—were armed with self-help manuals on the preparation for death. This generation would not be caught off guard when death came calling.

The Death of the Art of Dying

The *ars moriendi* body of literature dominated the European and (later) American cultural landscapes for hundreds of years, into the early twentieth century. But around the time that my patient Gertrude Capella was born, the art of dying began to give way to the art of living.

The shift was subtle. Whereas the *ars moriendi* taught that a person cultivated good life habits with a view to dying well, the early twentieth century came to focus solely on living well—death and dying be damned.

The economic growth of the Roaring Twenties promised a new way of life. More people drove cars, listened to radio, watched movies, and followed the glamorous lives of celebrities. Industry boomed, and the latest consumer goods became topics of conversation. Women made widows by World War I began to eschew traditional mourning practices. Women voted, and the young danced. A distinctively modern age had dawned.

Within medicine, a number of developments promised the extension of life and hinted at the possibility that death itself might one day die. In 1928, Alexander Fleming identified penicillin, which opened the door to a host of other infection-killing, life-prolonging antibiotics. By the 1950s, intensive-care units, mechanical ventilators, and cardiopulmonary resuscitation methods were successfully staving off death. And by the early 1960s, doctors were miraculously transplanting organs. With so much forward momentum, why ponder human finitude? It is no wonder that now, in her mid-nineties, Ms. Capella has given scant consideration to preparing for her death.

A colleague of mine once told me about his grandfather, a brilliantly skilled carpenter. He wielded his tools to create the most elegant furniture. Renowned for his artistry, he constructed massive wooden backdrops for church and pub alike. But as he grew older, he built for himself a simple wooden coffin—an act that his family found strange and somewhat morbid. But the grandfather countered that there was no reason to waste money on purchasing a coffin when he had the skill. Constructing his own coffin served as an exercise in reflecting on his finitude and inviting his family to do the same.

Those of us in the West today will fail to die well if we refuse to acknowledge that we are finite creatures. Some people have sought a technological solution to our collective ignorance of finitude, and smartphone applications have been developed to encourage the contemplation of mortality. At random times of day and night, subscribers to a service called WeCroak receive "invitations to stop and think about death." They are usually in the form of sage quotations, such as "The grave has no sunny corners." Although WeCroak adopts the plural pronoun "we," the reminders of finitude go to the cell phone of each individual. There is no *we* in its practical application.

If the legend of the victorious Roman general is anything to go by, we may in reality require others to remind us of our humanness. The Roman general, the memento mori, and even the *ars moriendi* show us that reckoning with finitude is a task for both individuals and communities.

But there is another group of people who must acknowledge finitude—doctors. In order for us to learn once again the art of dying well, medical professionals must acknowledge the limitations of the treatments and technologies on offer. If physicians continue to tempt patients with illusions of immortality through various life-prolonging procedures, they propagate deception and fail to equip patients to face wisely the final and arguably most important task of their lives. We will return to this in the last chapter.

The *ars moriendi* was never intended to be practiced by an individual in isolation. Just as each of us requires support from a community, so too can communities garner strength from gathering to support an individual's sickness. It is to the community that we now turn.

CHAPTER THREE

COMMUNITY

Juan Plaza and Ronald Rodriguez work in New York on behalf of an overlooked group: those who die alone. Officially, they are called investigators, but their business is really search and rescue. They search the homes of the friendless dead and rescue two sorts of items: objects to aid in the deceased's identification and valuables to auction off for the estate.

The authorities are usually summoned by the growing stench of decay. The fire department's paramedic pronounces the death, no matter how decomposed the body, and the police attempt to notify next of kin. If, after nine days, no relative comes forward, the case falls to a little-known agency named the Queens County Public Administrator. Each county in

New York City has a public administrator to handle the estates of the unaccompanied dead, and Mr. Plaza and Mr. Rodriguez work for Queens County.

Clad in hazmat suits, respiratory masks, and surgical shoe covers, they look as though they should be battling Ebola rather than rescuing the treasures of the dead. They open drawers, peer into medicine cabinets, and dig through closets. They collect watches and laptop computers, photographs, tax returns—anything that could identify next of kin. If ever there was a modern memento mori, this investigative work is it. All day long Plaza and Rodriguez are reminded that they too will die.

The journalist N. R. Kleinfield's *New York Times* article "The Lonely Death of George Bell" describes how Rodriguez and Plaza have been transformed by this work. The shadow cast by human finitude prompts Mr. Rodriguez to live each day fully, "like it's the last day," while Mr. Plaza has redoubled his efforts never to die alone. He regularly connects to his community of support. Each day he sends his friends inspirational electronic messages, so that when he fails to do so, they will assume he has died and come looking for his body. He does not want to end up like George Bell, who died alone and was not found until six days later.

Dying Alone or Dying Lonely?

Kleinfield describes George Bell's death as "lonely." Loneliness, however, is an emotional response to the state of being alone. We all spend some part of each day alone—showering, going to the toilet—but we are not in these instances lonely. Was Mr. Bell lonely? Kleinfield's account does not provide a satisfactory answer. Bell seems to have had one close friend, Frank Bertone, with whom he met regularly, including the week before he died. But Mr. Bertone reported that Bell never disclosed the details of his personal life. Bell also appears to have been a hoarder, and Kleinfield notes that hoarding is considered a mental disorder that can prompt "incoherent acts." Perhaps his symptoms did not include feelings of loneliness. We will never know.

It is entirely possible, however, that Kleinfield's title does not properly refer to Bell's experience of death at all. Perhaps it is we, the readers, who label as "lonely" the death of a man whose demise is announced by the smell of decomposing flesh. Like Juan Plaza, we fear dying alone, and the emotional response of fear prompts us to diagnose George Bell's as a lonely death.

Bell was not famous—"just another man," as Kleinfield puts it. He began investigating Bell's story because he wondered how, in an overcrowded metropolis like New York, people end up dying unnoticed and alone. His investigation and reporting somehow imbued Bell's life with meaning as well as served as a testimony to the lives and deaths of the many others who die unaccompanied in New York City each year.

But it is not just in New York. Two years after the *Times* ran Kleinfield's piece, it published an account of the same phenomenon on the other side of the globe: "A Generation in Japan Faces a Lonely Death." Through the story of the ninety-one-year-old widow Chieko Ito, the reporter, Norimitsu Onishi, describes the growing prevalence of lonely deaths in Japan's large apartment complexes, or *danchi*.

Mrs. Ito moved to the Tokiwadaira *danchi* shortly after World War II. This was a period of modernization and growth in Japan. The complex, with its 4,800 apartments in 171 matching buildings, offered the latest in household appliances: washing machines, televisions, and refrigerators. Mrs. Ito's husband boarded the train to Tokyo for work six days a week, and she herself taught at a preschool within the complex. The place was lively. Children swarmed through playgrounds and splashed through wading pools. Laughter and shrieks of delight drifted in through open apartment windows. All was bursting with life, that is, until those children grew up—and their parents grew old.

In 1992, Mrs. Ito's husband and daughter both died within a three-month period. She has one stepdaughter, but they seldom communicate. She has gradually outlived close friends, acquaintances, and siblings. "I've been lonely for twenty-five years," she is quoted as saying. "They're the ones to blame for dying. I'm angry."

Not only do many of the aging *danchi* dwellers die alone, but their dying is lonely—they lack community. "We are fools to depend upon the society of our fellow men," the seventeenth-century French mathematician Blaise Pascal once claimed. "They will not aid us; we shall die alone."

The first lonely death in Mrs. Ito's *danchi* came to public attention in the year 2000. The man had died three years earlier, but no one had realized, because his expenses had been deducted automatically from his bank account each month. When his savings were exhausted, the authorities came to his apartment to investigate. They found a skeleton stripped of its flesh by maggots and beetles. Since then, such deaths have become more common. In the summer of 2017, a popular Japanese magazine reported an estimated four thousand lonely deaths a week.

Mrs. Ito is so afraid of being discovered dead and alone that she has asked a neighbor who lives in the building opposite hers to check her window daily. If Mrs. Ito fails to open her paper screen one morning, it means that she has died, and the neighbor should summon the authorities. In exchange for this service, Mrs. Ito sends the neighbor a gift every summer.

The tragedy of this situation is not lost on the Japanese. With half the residents of Tokiwadaira above the age of sixty-five, community leaders have created a network of volunteers to visit tenants who appear particularly vulnerable. Residents have also organized monthly lunches for those who live alone. The goal, Onishi explains, is to build community and combat isolation. Indeed, some success has been achieved. Lonely deaths in Tokiwadaira have dropped from about fifteen per year in the early 2000s to ten per year in 2017. For those ten, and for the countless others like them, a service has developed that will clean out their apartments. A similar service emptied the contents of Mr. Bell's apartment after his body was discovered.

Rehearsing for Death

Whether in New York City or Tokyo, dying lonely feels wrong. No one, we insist, should die alone. This instinct is probably as old as the human race. Indeed, for most of human history, dying has more typically been a community affair. Care of the dying, death, and funerals unite communities in ways that little else can.

Together with the acknowledgment of human finitude, the role of community was central to the *ars moriendi*. As discussed in the previous chapter, a substantial portion of the original *ars moriendi* text provided specific instructions to friends and family gathered at the deathbed. Not only were they to intercede with petitions and prayers on behalf of the dying, they were expected to take the opportunity to examine their own readiness for death. Everyone had work to do to prepare for death. For the living, that work extended beyond the deathbed into daily life.

In his monumental volume on the history of Western attitudes toward death, the French historian Philippe Ariès asserts that a public aspect of death was customary in the West until the late nineteenth century. When the death bell tolled, community members gathered. In fact, Ariès reports, so many people flocked to the bedside of the dying that "hygienically minded doctors of the late eighteenth century" decried the practice and attempted to persuade the masses to stay away. This effort failed, however, and, according to Ariès, the convention in western Europe continued to be such that even a stranger could visit the dying once the so-called last rites had been administered.

The *ars moriendi* literary genre sometimes characterized dying as a drama in which *moriens* (the dying person) is the protagonist and all other members of the patient's community, from youngest to oldest, play supporting roles. The idea is that those in attendance at the deathbed could rehearse their roles in this familial drama while still young and healthy, in anticipation of their own future role as *moriens*. Rehearsing made it easier to sustain a supportive community once death hovered. When someone died, there would be no guessing about what one should do or say.

The *ars moriendi* was practiced widely in the West for more than five hundred years. Ariès tells the story of the seventeenth-century French courtier Madame de Montespan to dramatize the way the *moriens* and her supportive community interacted.

Madame de Montespan reportedly feared dying alone far more than she feared death itself. Beautiful and fiercely witty, she charmed her way into the court of King Louis XIV of France. Although she was married with children, she became the king's *maîtresse-en-titre*, or official chief mistress, and bore him seven children. An excellent conversationalist, she kept herself abreast of political events and spoke her mind, winning the attention and admiration of many prominent figures of her day. She was not France's official queen, but her contemporaries often considered her the "reigning beauty," given her profound influence on the court.

In death, as in life, Madame de Montespan surrounded her-self with people. As she lay dying, she insisted that the bed curtains remain open. If the women attending her dozed off, she woke them up and encouraged them to participate in some manner—perhaps by talking, grooming, or eating. She insisted on directing the activity about her, even as her own ability to participate waned.

When the *maîtresse-en-titre* realized that she was about to die, she followed the *ars moriendi* instructions. Ariès writes: "She summoned all her servants, 'down to the lowest one,' asked their forgiveness, confessed her sins, and presided, as was the custom, over the ceremony of her own death." Ma-dame de Montespan was the protagonist of the great drama of her life and death. Her servants and attendants had re-hearsed their roles. They knew how to provide a community of support to Madame, while also practicing for their own dying.

Harvey and Sara

Like Madame de Montespan, we may not want to die alone, but most of us would not wish for a return to the fullness of *ars moriendi* practice, where countless strangers and acquain-tances visited the dying. Just as few women choose to share the experience of childbirth with more than a select group, so too few of us wish to make the messiness of death a public spectacle.

But we want somebody there when we die, and it is worth rehearsing for the inevitable in community now—while we have our wits about us and are able-bodied. Community does not materialize instantly at a deathbed; it must be cultivated over a lifetime.

My patient Sara Weinberg, a natural storyteller, told me one day of how she and her husband anticipated and in some sense "rehearsed" for his death. In what follows I have attempted to capture Sara's narrative.

It was their fifty-first wedding anniversary, and Sara spent the day sitting at Harvey's bedside in the hospital. His health had been shaky for years, the degree and duration of the shakiness surpassed only, perhaps, by that of their marriage. Fifty-one *long* years. But they had made it! They were still together. To celebrate that remarkable accomplishment, Sara sat faithfully, unusually quietly, in the institutional-grade, faux-leather chair that had been placed alongside Harvey's hospital bed. They didn't say much. After fifty-one years all had been said. Or shouted. What was left?

I had been Sara's primary-care doctor for a long time, and I knew that her marital accomplishment had not come easily. "Haavey"—as she called him—had strong opinions. On everything. And he let them be known. But Sara wasn't one to have her own views overruled, so they quarreled regularly.

After nearly a half century of marriage, she had announced at her appointment with me one day that she thought they needed marriage counseling. "I just can't take it anymore," she explained. Harvey wasn't mean or abusive or anything particularly alarming. He was just, well—*Harvey*. And he was becoming more and more *Harvey* with age. What was she to do? We devoted our office visit to discussing options, and I sent her home with a list of marriage counselors and suggestions for small interventions, such as finding a reason to get out of the house by herself each day.

They had gone for counseling, she got out of the house, and things improved.

Sara had accompanied her husband to each of his many doctor's visits. As a result, she had become well acquainted with his primary-care doctor. In light of Harvey's declining health, the doctor and Sara had spoken regularly of getting the proverbial house in order. She had put together a folder of all their important legal documents. Their children were on speed dial. They had practiced just what to do when he died.

Sara left the hospital on the night of their anniversary feeling content. Harvey had been sick for so long, but sickness was part of life—and of death. They had spent a wonderful day together, which somehow made the five decades of hardship seem worthwhile.

When she received a call from the hospital several hours later, it didn't really come as a surprise. "Mrs. Weinberg? I am sorry to tell you this, but Mr. Weinberg has passed. Can you please come back to the hospital?"

He had died alone in the hospital. Perhaps Harvey thought it was better this way, she reasoned. Maybe he was waiting for her to leave before he relaxed his grip on life. Sometimes people do that. And besides, she had just been with him, so it wasn't as if his had been a lonely death. She changed back into her clothes, picked up the folder, and drove herself to the hospital.

She parked the car and walked toward the hospital's front doors. He had been sick a long time, and she felt that strange combination of sadness and relief—more like pepper and salt than oil and water—a mixture of feelings that often overwhelms the recently bereaved. The elevator doors entombed her as she rode to the fifth floor. It was one o'clock in the morning, and for the first time in decades she was alone.

The hospital ward was quiet and dark as she walked down the hall toward Harvey's room. Somehow the hallway felt much longer now. Had they moved him farther down the ward? She took note, as she walked, of sounds emerging from other patients' rooms: sporadic snoring, relentless beeping, an occasional delirious patient calling out. Death had brought into relief the little reminders of life that remained in the dark night.

She paused outside his room. What would he look like? Would he be cold if she touched him? Would he look peaceful? She could see around the doorway that his bedside light shone down on him. Maybe the nurses were busy doing paperwork at the bedside. Or maybe they always leave the lights on over the deceased, like an angelic glow.

Sara mustered all her courage and walked into the room.

"Hullo, Sara!" a voice boomed.

"Hi, Haavey," she said. "What are you doing here?"

"It's the middle of the night. I was about to ask you the same thing!" Harvey replied.

He looked just the same as he had several hours earlier: very much alive.

The nurse manager, floor nurse, and doctor arrived a moment later. There had been a terrible mistake. The neighboring patient had died, and in the fluster that accompanies a failed attempt at resuscitating the dead, the poor junior doctor tasked with notifying the next of kin had dialed the wrong number. He felt positively wretched for having committed such a blunder and practically threw himself at Sara's feet with remorse.

It did not bother Sara. She had lived through worse.

The hospital administration followed up with a shipment of potted flowers. Sara put them on her dining-room table beside the folder of legal documents. She determined that the plants would stay alive as long as Harvey did.

Sara was a schoolteacher famous for her sense of humor, and she added this account to her collection of stories. When I saw her several months later, we laughed about it. She gave me permission to tell her story with a few identifiers changed.

"When the hospital called to tell me Haavey died, I didn't call my son right away. First I called my boyfriend and told him to chill the champagne." (There was no boyfriend, but she thought it made for a good twist.) She went on. "The only thing worse than going to the hospital in the middle of the night because your husband's died is showing up and finding out he hasn't!" We laughed again.

Marriage had its challenges, but she loved Harvey. They were a team. He was her closest community.

Commitment to Community

What should we expect of our communities? Harvey and Sara
struggled together for decades. That is often the case with family and close friends. Our communities of support do not have
to be perfect, but they should feel hospitable. We should feel
safe among those who love us and have committed to looking
after us.

Some of the *ars moriendi* texts warned against permitting
contentious individuals to visit the deathbed. They argued that
the possibility of dying well could be thwarted by the presence
of bitter, hostile, or avaricious temperaments. Although there
is some wisdom here, I suspect that it should not be taken as
an absolute. In my medical practice I have witnessed time and
time again that, as death approaches, the most antagonistic
of relationships can experience healing. Dying can create an
opportunity for reconciliation that might not otherwise be
possible.

Although the deathbed offers a chance for community
members to converge in deeper and more meaningful ways,
the *ars moriendi* did not intend that community building occur only at the point of death. Relationship building as well
as the preparation for death were meant to take place over the
course of a lifetime.

Community helps us to clarify our sense of self and what
we value most. Many of my patients have described how illness
and dying have caused their worlds to become smaller, but also
more meaningful. As they become less able to travel, leave the

house, or even get out of bed, they find that they don't miss their previous level of activity as much as they thought they would. Instead, they discover new delights. Lingering over a favorite meal with family and close friends brings a deeper joy. So too does the opportunity to sit together with a loved one and observe the changing color of a room as evening approaches. The prospect of Harvey's death made Sara realize how grateful she was for his companionship.

Community can also encourage us to invest further in what we value. Some of my patients continue to be very active even as they are dying. Some have thrown their energy into social causes. Others have devoted themselves more deeply to their faith communities. Still others have created projects that they know will outlive them and continue to represent their passions and commitments. In all cases, the ideas are conceived and realized within the context of community.

Communities also aid in making sense of life's big questions of meaning and purpose. Why am I here? What does life mean? What happens when we die? Whether religious or not, most of us come from communities that offer some sort of basic response to these fundamental questions. Engaging those responses and accepting, rejecting, or modifying them is part of what shapes our identities in relationship to our communities.

Community can also help the dying in completing the tasks necessary to die well. The *ars moriendi* exhorted the dying and those at the bedside to attend to physical and spiritual matters of import—writing their wills and making peace with God. This was Madame de Montespan's practice. She invited her servants to participate in her dying process, inadvertently compelling them to acknowledge their own finitude. And at the very end she conducted the final tasks of dying well by gathering them, confessing her faults, and asking their forgiveness.

Some of the practices within the context of hospice and palliative medicine today bear marked similarities to *ars moriendi* counsel. The palliative-care doctor Ira Byock suggests that, in addition to arranging financial and legal matters, the dying should ask themselves about other affairs, such as, "Are your relationships also 'in order'?" Byock notes that hospice provides a model for "relationship completion" by encouraging the dying to say five phrases: "I forgive you," "Forgive me," "Thank you," "I love you," and "Goodbye"—basic instructions that are similar to the approach taken by Madame de Montespan in her dying.

Three Levels of Community

As a medical doctor who thinks a lot about preparing for death, I suggest that we might consider community as existing on three levels. Community's foundation is, first, among *family* and close friends, and much of what has just been discussed pertains to this basic level of intimate community. But the notion of community extends further, to society more broadly, and even to the biomedical community. The *societal community* might include all those who support the aging and infirm, from ride-share programs to Meals on Wheels to the network of volunteers visiting the lonely elderly in Japan's *danchi*. The *biomedical community* includes the teams of social workers, chaplains, therapists, doctors, nurses, and other health-care professionals who accompany particular patients as illness takes hold and death draws near.

When I think about community existing on these three levels—familial, societal, biomedical—my patient Diana Atwood Johnson comes to mind. I met Diana a number of years ago after she was first diagnosed with a terminal lung disease. At that time, she was given several months to live.

I had been wrapping up work on an academic book on the *ars moriendi* the day she first burst into my office. "I'm dying. I know I'm dying. I need you to help me through this," she had said, just moments before hurriedly pouring out her entire life story. She was facing her finitude squarely, and this prompted her to reflect on her community.

As we spoke, she began to speculate about her possible decline over the months ahead, and she named all those who would partner with her. She would rely on a tight group of friends who could help her attend wisely to death and "consider its excesses in light of its deprivation, its beauty in light of its decay." As I had then written, "Community helps us to recognize frail hopes and joys that surface in the midst of adversity. Relationships clarify the goods that we value and the ends to which we orient ourselves."

Nearly five years later, by the time I was writing this book, Diana had far outlived her initial prognosis. But her autoimmune lung condition continued in hot pursuit, and she remained well aware that it was only a matter of time. While I was writing this chapter, she was admitted with breathing difficulties to our hospital's step-down unit, which provides higher-intensity care than a regular medical ward but slightly less than an intensive-care unit.

After four and a half years of meeting in my clinic *outside* the hospital, it felt ominous to see her there, with a life-saving breathing mask strapped to her face. I entered her hospital room and took a seat beside her recliner. "Hey, Diana." My voice was quiet. "Just wanted to swing by and say hello." I wasn't visiting her in any formal capacity; I had simply stopped by as her friend and primary-care doctor, because she was so sick. We both recognized that the circumstances were graver than they had ever been before. I was unsure of what to say next when her phone rang.

She picked up the phone, inspected the name on caller ID, and said that she would return the call later. She had just had two friends stop by her hospital room, and this friend would not mind waiting. We spoke for a few minutes, and the phone rang again, a different friend. We tried to resume the conversation, when her iPad announced that a message had arrived. And so it went. Diana's *familial* community was in place, mobilized to help her in this next stage of her illness and decline.

She had also been expanding her *societal* community. In recent months she had been meeting regularly with her minister. In addition, she had been working with an eldercare adviser to set up all of the actors slightly further afield who would enable her to remain in her own home, if possible, as her health declined. She was planning for everything that was beyond the scope of what her community of family and friends could provide.

We also talked about her *biomedical* community—her new doctor, her old doctors, the respiratory therapists, physicians' assistants, and others who formed her medical team. Diana recognized that all of these community members were crucial both for the ongoing management of her disease and for her dying well. She understood that her lungs were weakening and that borrowed time on a mechanical ventilator would offer no lasting fix. She wanted neither cardiac resuscitation, were her heart to stop, nor intubation with a breathing tube. My last task as her primary-care doctor that night was to speak with the physician's assistant outside her hospital room to make sure that her "Do Not Resuscitate" orders were in place.

I marveled at Diana as I walked out of the hospital. She had taken to heart the *ars moriendi*. And here she was, more than four years since our first meeting, fully aware of her finitude and with community in place to die well. She was daily practicing the art, and by all reasonable assessments she would indeed die well.

If only this could be the case for more of us.

Salmon on Silver

After I visited her that night in the hospital, Diana spent some six weeks in two different rehabilitation facilities before being discharged home on December 21. She was readmitted to our hospital the day after Christmas.

I had not had the winter holidays off work for more than a decade. This year I received a break, so I committed to traveling with family. Diana and I kept in touch regularly by email while I was on the road. On December 28, she ended her letter this way:

> Anyway, the bad news according to Dr. K . . . I need to move on to palliative and hospice care. Do not pass go. . . . Their plan is to fix me up enough to go home to die. That will probably be next week. No knowing, but I'm safe here, which I haven't felt anywhere for a while. Dr. K seems to be straightforward enough, maybe a little harsh like D, but informative and will talk about anything if I ask. Reminds me of a chapter in your book. . . . It's tough news the closer it gets, but I have so much love and support. I think their hearts might break more than mine.
> Enough. Tears use up oxygen.
> xoxo
> Diana

It was New Year's Day when I was again able to access the electronic medical record. With record low temperatures outside and a warm laptop on my knees, I started the new year the way I would predictably finish it—catching up on my patients' health news. I scanned the dozens of test results, patient emails, and notes from subspecialists searching for updates on Diana, who had not written in a couple of days.

Buried at the end of a doctor's note from New Year's Eve was mention of a discussion with her "familial community" about changing the focus of her care from cure to comfort. Diana was dying. That sinister lung-destroying disease had no intention of relinquishing its grip on her life.

I began scouring her doctors' notes in earnest. I found a message in the electronic health record from a colleague. Diana's breathing had become so labored that the medical team had started a morphine drip to ease her distress. She had not liked how the morphine dulled her mentally and had previously refused it. But she knew that morphine would thwart the feeling of suffocation. By accepting the drip, she was accepting death's imminence.

I picked up the phone and called my colleague. "How is she doing?" I asked.

"She just passed. Some of her friends are at the bedside."

I put the phone down, said goodbye to my family, and drove straight to the hospital.

Entering Diana's hospital room, I surveyed the scene. Her body lay in the bed, waxy and firm. Life takes its leave so quickly.

Surrounding the bed were many of those who loved her most—old friends, her minister, a fellow birdwatcher. Even in death, she was not alone. She had told each of us stories about the others. Although we had just met, it felt like a reunion of old friends.

I went to the bed and stroked her shoulder. It seemed like the right thing to do—laying hands on the body of a person I had examined countless times before. I was consoling myself through the same touch I use to console others. But this time I was the only one who could feel the touch.

Her minister kissed her brow. "She wouldn't let 2017 take her. No, she wouldn't," he said.

Overcome, I burst into tears.

"You look like you need a hug," someone said. I turned around to find the receiving arms of a woman who had just entered the room. It turned out that she was one of Diana's closest friends as well as her health-care decision-maker. Janie embraced me as if time had stopped.

Without a hint of awkwardness, we stepped apart and introduced ourselves. Then all of us in the room began to trade stories. That's when I learned about the salmon on a silver platter.

One of Diana's greatest grievances during her protracted stays in the rehabilitation facilities was the food. Just before Christmas, she had emailed me a discursive reflection on her finitude, followed by a lament. "If I never have to eat institutional food again, it will be too soon. Oh my goodness, it was bad." We could not fix her disease, but maybe we could do something about the food.

So Janie did. On Christmas Eve, Janie and her husband made the nearly two-hour drive to Diana's home with "the best smoked salmon in Greenwich" on a silver platter. Janie had browned her own mini-toasts and arranged all the fixings.

Diana, of course, relished every bite. The Feast of the Seven Fishes could not have come close.

On the eve of New Year's Eve, when the sand in Diana's hourglass had nearly emptied, Janie repeated the gift—salmon on a silver platter, linen tablecloth, china dishes, and goblets. This time they dined in the hospital. Diana's last supper.

One Dies Alone

Not everyone has such a robust community. Stories like those of George Bell and Chieko Ito remind us that people do better when they are less lonely. People are meant to live in community. We are relational creatures.

Some of the hardest deaths for those of us who work in health care occur when we cannot locate any family or friends for a dying patient. We even have a term for them— "unbefriended." Who can speak to the values or beliefs of the unbefriended? Who will make their medical decisions? In such instances, we partner with social workers and care coordinators in the unified mission of locating next of kin or *anyone* who might be equipped to speak on behalf of the patient.

I once cared for a woman who had recently relocated to my city. She was widowed and estranged from her only daughter. She had previously been healthy, but in the months prior to our visit her memory seemed to have declined—some sort of rapidly progressing dementia. In short, she was losing her mind, and she was all alone.

Given the severity of her decline, I spent a significant part of our visit trying to determine if there was anyone, any person in the world, whom she wanted me to contact on her behalf. This woman needed people to support her in her frailty. I had no doubt that my most important task as her new primary-care doctor was to help assemble those people. Eventually I was able to establish a community of old friends who promised to keep tabs on her. I hoped she would die more like Madame de Montespan than George Bell.

Writing in the 1970s, Philippe Ariès concludes his discussion of Madame de Montespan's deathbed community with poignant words that still apply today:

Death was always public. Hence the profound significance of Pascal's remark that one dies alone, for at that time one was never physically alone at the moment of death. Today his statement has lost its impact, for one has a very good chance of literally dying alone, in a hospital room.

Or in a Japanese *danchi*. Or in a New York City apartment.

CHAPTER FOUR

CONTEXT

Does it matter where we die? Many of us have a vision of dying at home surrounded by those we love. That's certainly what I have always imagined for myself. But if dying ends in death, can we say that our physical location, once we are dead, matters to us any longer? Dead bodies don't care whether they lie in a bedroom or a refrigerated morgue.

What really distresses us is not the idea of being dead in a hospital; it is the idea of *dying* there, of what we experience *before* we go. Who wouldn't shudder at the thought of languishing in a sterile medical ward, too sick to escape, imprisoned by illness, dependent on futuristic machines, at the mercy of an anonymous throng of health-care professionals? I have taken care of far too many terminal patients to wish for the same sort of exit.

The problem, however, is the haziness of the line between slow physical decline requiring frequent hospital readmissions and the *ultimate* admission, that hospital stay from which we never escape. We depend on doctors to stave off death, yet tell ourselves we will go home if nothing else can be done. Indeed, some 80 percent of Americans prefer to die at home when possible.

Why, then, do we want to die at home? George Bell and some of the *danchi*-dwelling Japanese died at home, but they died unnoticed and alone. My patient Diana attempted to go home to die, but ultimately surrendered to a hospital death. For Diana, who lived alone, the hospital proved hospitable. There she felt safe and cared for.

For most of us, the home stands as a constant in a rapidly changing world. The home is uniquely ours, where we exist, where we can simply be. Although the average American moves about eleven times, there remains a certain constancy to home life—pets and people, to be sure, but also *that* chair, *that* painting, *that* perennial plant. The home is where we feast and celebrate, weep and mourn, sit and stare. If the outside world demands that we be poised and professional, home accepts us at our most authentic. Home embraces us, silently consoling us with the knowledge that we belong to *this* home. Why would we die anywhere else?

Childbed to Tree of the Dead

Birth and death bracket a life. The trajectory is birth, life, death. Our sense of belonging to a place correlates with the extent to which this trajectory occurs in a single location. Those who are born, live, and die in the same place call that place "home." But this is increasingly unusual. For the rootless, "home" might be the place where they spend the majority of their days or their most recent days. Or "home" may be harder to pin down. Some of us, myself included, call multiple places "home."

The philosopher Martin Heidegger famously wrote about the traditional peasant farmhouse in Germany's Black Forest. It was a dwelling designed to meet the needs over time of families who lived in a community that was rooted in a specific place. The peasant belonged to the house, which belonged to the landscape, which belonged to the beginning. The peasant could not die anywhere else.

Heidegger saw the farmhouse as ordered by the "simple oneness" of all that is seen and unseen—earth, heaven, mortals, divinities. The slope of the mountain shelters the south-facing house from wind. The meadows adjoin a spring-fed water source. The wide overhanging roof withstands the weight of heavy snow and shields the rooms inside from winter storms. Heidegger was not a religious man, but he saw in this arrangement a connection to the cosmos, a bridge to the wider world, and a relationship to the land, the cycle of seasons, and the elements.

That same earthy-ethereal "simple oneness" also affects the interior of the farm hut. Heidegger describes an "altar corner behind the community table" meant for religious iconography. The bedchamber, he writes, made space for "the hallowed places of childbed and the 'tree of the dead'—for that is what they call a coffin there: the *Totenbaum*—and in this way it designed for the different generations under one roof the character of their journey through time."

The farmhouse itself symbolizes the cycle of life. The home makes provision for both cradle and coffin, the recently born and the recently deceased—together under the watchful eye of the religious icon in the altar corner. From birth to death, the peasant belongs here, her existence reified by an occupied seat at the community table—her death, by an empty chair.

Heidegger doubtless romanticizes the farmhouse, an attitude rendered disquieting by his affiliation with Nazism. His own Black Forest house, which he used as a sort of philosopher's retreat, contained neither cradle nor coffin. His occupancy was always temporary—he would not die there.

But if we set aside Heidegger himself and ponder only the description of the farmhouse, we can appreciate how intertwined our homes are with our very being. Imagine generations of family members inhabiting the same place or even the same house. In such circumstances, who wouldn't want to die at home? Although our lives now are considerably more mobile, there remains a sense in which we belong to our homes. And even if, for whatever reason, we cannot die at home, we may wish to die surrounded by the people and possessions that best evoke the feeling of home.

Why, then, do the majority of Americans die in institutions, such as hospitals, nursing homes, extended-care facilities, and hospices? Why does only one in five Americans die at home?

Domestic Medicine

Hospitals began in the West as places of hospitality for wayfarers and the poor. Basil of Caesarea, a fourth-century Greek bishop, established what many consider to have been the predecessor to the modern Western hospital. He constructed a massive city-size complex, the Basiliad, just outside Caesarea, in what today is Israel. It began in 369 as a sort of soup kitchen, and by 372 it housed medical professionals who cared for the sick.

The Basiliad's doctors treated many diseases including leprosy, which was ordinarily shunned. Its grounds included housing for the poor, a hospice for the dying, a school for orphans, and lodging for travelers. All care—medical, physical, educational—was provided free of charge, funded by charitable donations. Within a century, many similar hospitals were established throughout the Roman Empire.

Despite Basil's extraordinary success, most people over the subsequent fifteen hundred years died at home. In Philippe Ariès's collection of nearly one thousand years' worth of stories of death, he describes how "a whole little society of neighbors and friends" shared the "burden of care and unpleasantness." The lower classes and rural poor developed the most extensive care networks, but middle-class circles also relied on them. Wealthier families were attended by their servants. Regardless of socioeconomic class, the dying person continued to be the central actor in that great *ars moriendi* drama; only the most destitute resorted to going to hospitals to die.

In his 1984 Pulitzer Prize–winning book, the sociologist Paul Starr corroborates Ariès's account through his description of the transformation of specifically American medicine from 1760 onward. Starr describes the family in early American society as the "natural locus of most care of the sick." It was the women of the household who dried the medicinal herbs and stocked the home-remedy cabinet. In cases of severe illness, they relied upon older, more experienced women in the community for counsel and assistance. Rarely did they think of calling a doctor.

Colonial newspapers and almanacs circulated medical advice to augment oral tradition. Health practitioners, such as the doctor William Buchan in Scotland, began to publish lay guides describing home treatments. Buchan was a member of Scotland's exclusive Royal College of Physicians, but he considered his colleagues obstacles to progress. He thought that they should share their knowledge rather than keep their discoveries to themselves.

Buchan valued the medical profession, but he also believed

that the profession had nothing to lose if ordinary people could understand it. That is why he published, in 1769, his work *Domestic Medicine*. The book's lengthy subtitle explains clearly its purpose: *The Family Physician: Being an attempt to render the Medical Art more generally useful, by shewing people what is in their own power both with respect to the Prevention and Cure of Diseases.* With explanations of diseases, treatments, and prevention at their fingertips, laypeople quickly embraced this guide to the art of living well, an accompaniment to the art of dying well. Buchan's book remained popular for more than a century and was reprinted in the United States in at least thirty editions.

Many doctors in Europe and the United States subsequently published similar guides, securing the home's role as the preferred site for care of the sick and dying.

The Hospital: Horror or Hope?

It wasn't simply that self-sufficient Americans were capable of handling the sick and dying at home. Members of civilized society would never have dreamed of setting foot in hospitals—those charitable institutions for the unbefriended poor, lonely wayfarers, or isolated elderly. But hospitals would not forever remain "places of dreaded impurity and exiled human wreckage," to borrow Starr's phrase. They were to become beacons of hope, "awesome citadels of science and bureaucratic order."

This shift occurred toward the end of the nineteenth century. Although European hospitals, from the eighteenth century onward, played important roles in medical research and education, the same was not true in the United States. Starting around 1870, American hospitals also started assuming a more prominent role in medical education and practice.

Medicine began to organize, professionalize, and compete in financial markets. Buchan's domestic medicine now became hospital medicine, concentrating both expertise and expensive equipment. Starr explains:

> What drove this transformation was not simply the advance of science, important though that was, but the demands and example of an industrializing capitalist society, which brought larger numbers of people into urban centers, detached them from traditions of self-sufficiency, and projected ideals of specialization and technical competence.

The hospital, which was once a place of dreaded horror, had now become "a workplace for the production of health." Doctors could now offer so much more than comfort; they could cure.

Progress and promise defined the mood. Industrialization brought steady employment. Members of rural families moved to urban centers to pursue work, and this migration weakened ties to larger communities that could support workers who fell ill. Moreover, small city apartments lacked space to care for the sick. With the hospital's growing list of therapeutic offerings, it presented a reasonable alternative.

Starr devotes hundreds of pages to describing this transformation, a riveting story that I commend to curious readers. But for our purposes, what is worth highlighting is the rapid growth of hospitals in the United States. In 1873, there existed fewer than two hundred hospitals; by 1910 there were more than four thousand and by 1920 more than six thousand, which is slightly greater than the number of hospitals today.

Within a half century, hospitals lost their stigma and rapidly proliferated. And with urbanization, more people than ever lived in their proximity. Americans became increasingly reliant on hospital services. But the question that remains unanswered is this: If we feel most comforted in our homes, why then would we want to die in a hospital?

The Rescue Fantasy

The sickness that leads to death is for many life's greatest tragedy. Many times I have sat with patients who have received a death sentence and who have pleaded with me to review the test results one more time. *Is the specialist correct? Am I really dying?* As I reread the data on the computer screen, I feel the patient's eyes press into me.

I once had a patient with a very bizarre set of symptoms. I met with him monthly for years, poring over his photocopy-paper boxes of old medical records and ordering what was doubtless hundreds of thousands of dollars of tests. I watched him experiment methodically with diet, environment, and exposure—efforts to identify what could be making him waste away. I sent him to specialists and even admitted him to the hospital to expedite an intensive workup. Each time we met, I felt his imploring gaze. *Doctor, do something. I am dying. Rescue me.*

Before a patient becomes a patient in that sixteenth-century sense of "recipient of the doctor's agency," the patient first experiences a health crisis. When disaster strikes or death threatens, patients look to doctors to save them. The bioethicist Albert Jonsen says: "Our moral response to the imminence of death demands that we rescue the doomed. We throw a rope to the drowning, rush into burning buildings to snatch the entrapped, dispatch teams to search for the snowbound." Jonsen then makes a critical pivot: "This rescue morality spills over into medical care"—an obligation he calls the "rule of rescue."

The hospital brims with rescue techniques—replacement organs, kidney machines, lung ventilators. Physicians try to follow the principle that the benefit of the intervention should outweigh the burden. This calculus endures until death looms, and then a compulsion to rescue overrides rationality. It no longer matters whether a medical intervention causes harm and produces poor outcomes. As rescuer, the doctor feels duty-bound to save the patient.

Doctors love to be rescuers, heroes who descend from on high to fight evil disease and liberate patients in distress. It is part of our common mythology. The bioethicist Howard

Brody says that this "rescue fantasy is a power trip: it envisions the physician having the power to snatch the patient from the jaws of death." Is not this image, after all, frequently part of doctors' attraction to the practice of medicine?

For their part, patients seek a rescuer to release them from their life-destroying maladies. When life itself is at stake, patients rarely want doctors who take the cost-effective, risk-balancing, rational approach. We are simply not wired to think this way. We want a doctor-savior who will stop at nothing. Timidity is not welcome where death lurks.

The physician's compulsion to rescue fuels the patient's burning desire to be rescued, which again stokes the doctor's rescue fantasy. The result is precisely the sort of medicalized dying described in Chapter One, when Amit and I attempted to resuscitate the dying Mr. Turner three times in a single night.

The Indecency of Death

We might summarize our story thus far as follows. For most of recorded history, people have died in their homes. In the fourth-century West, patrons began to build forerunners to the modern hospital, but these hospitals existed primarily to care for the poor and marginalized. Any integrated member of society could rely on care from community members in sickness and death. In due course, however, industrialization lured people out of their communities to the cities. Technological advances made new medical treatments and cures available.

Hospitals became the locus for care of the city-dwelling sick and for the dissemination of life-saving techniques. Doctors became rescuers.

But there was something else. Not only did hospitals entice with medicine and procedure; they also offered a welcome respite to families and community members saddled with the burden of caring for the sick and dying. The work has always been thankless and difficult—lifting weakened bodies, dressing foul-smelling wounds, washing debris from folds and crevices, assisting with toileting whether the infirm can rise from bed or not.

Even when the body is strong, the mind can fail and personality can change, causing the most devoted family member to become overwhelmed. My colleague, the physician-writer Marjorie Rosenthal, has described her own father's early-onset dementia and the toll this exacted on her family, especially her mother. As her mother assumed around-the-clock care of her father, Rosenthal grew worried by notable changes in her. She gave her mother a copy of a novel she was sure to love, but was shocked by what came next. "I was speechless when she gave it back to me and told me she couldn't concentrate long enough to read it." Endless caregiving, especially in isolation, has a negative impact on the caregiver's health. It can raise blood pressure, disrupt sleep, and trigger anxiety and depression.

One day, Rosenthal's father wandered into his neighbor's apartment, complaining that the woman with whom he lived made him clean all the time. Later, Rosenthal reminded him, "Dad, that's Mom you're living with. Your wife." He had no recollection of his forty-five years of marriage. Caring for him had become more taxing, and the family began to set in motion plans for him to move into a long-term residential care facility.

More than sixteen million Americans provide uncompensated care for people with Alzheimer's and other dementias. In 2018 dollars, this is estimated to be nearly $234 billion worth of services. And this is just for dementia. Were we to include unpaid care for people with end-stage cancers, heart failure, and lung disease, the burden would be substantially greater. It's no wonder that one-fifth of those caring for the elderly report that their health has deteriorated because of the work. And it's no wonder that when financially feasible, we look to professional surrogates to assume the labor—and the unpleasantness.

Prior to the rise of hospitals, families had cared for the sick and dying because no other alternative existed. But those under duress have always longed for relief. By the twentieth century, health-care institutions provided it. In addition to dispensing antibiotics and staffing ICUs, health-care professionals would now care for the sick and dying. This shift cemented hospitals, in Ariès's words, as "the scene of the normal death, expected and accepted by medical personnel."

Hideous sickness and indecent death had been relegated to the institution. If death had once been public and copulation taboo, the tide was turning. Death came to replace sex as the ultimate "unmentionable." In 1955, the English anthropologist Geoffrey Gorer labeled this phenomenon the "pornography of death." Death was sequestered from public view and dismissed as a subject of polite conversation.

Doctors failed to mention it. Families failed to witness it. The hospital promised to conquer it.

Dying in the Hospital—the Upshot

So we have moved from the coffin and cradle–equipped farmhouse to death in the hospital. A host of forces—cultural, economic, technological—conspired to establish sterile standardized institutions run by strangers as the default location for death. Today Americans are more comfortable discussing drug use and safe sex with their children than discussing preparation for death with their terminally ill parents. With the question of the *ars moriendi* ever before us, we must ask: Can there be any art to this sort of dying? The answer, I suggest, is yes. I arrive at this conclusion because of my patients.

Two of my patients—adult daughter and elderly father— planned an extended holiday to Tuscany. Samuel Loeb was in his early eighties, and although his heart had been tuned up several times, he was in relatively good shape. He had no reason not to travel, and besides, wine is supposed to be good for the heart. Italian health care, should he need it, would be able to address any concerns.

But the holiday took a dreadful turn. Mr. Loeb developed an infection, and his heart could not endure the resulting stress. It started to give way, and his lungs followed suit. His daughter Mandy took him to a hospital in Rome, where he was promptly admitted to intensive care and put on life support.

Because of time-zone differences, transatlantic pauses on the telephone, and a lack of access to his Italian medical record, I felt helpless. Everything his daughter told me sounded ominous. I encouraged her to extend her stay abroad, if possible.

Mandy did this several times. But she also arranged to have Mr. Loeb flown back to New York City on a medical jet, where he was directly admitted to the ICU under the care of his own cardiologist of thirty years. As she told me later, he wisely purchased travel insurance, which covered the medical jet, when he bought his plane ticket.

After nearly four weeks of intensive care on two continents, Mr. Loeb's infection rebounded, and he succumbed. When Mandy gave me the news, she said something else that stuck with me. "I am grateful that he was able to fly back to New York, because it was 'home,' and it was important to him. He was alert enough to know that he was back, and that gives me some comfort." Home—as country of origin, or country of residence, or place where the nursing staff speak to you in your own language, or where Medicare covers your hospitalization. *Home* can mean so much more than *house*.

My patient Diana died in the hospital but still experienced an art of dying, an *ars moriendi*. She outlived her prognosis by years and thus had ample time to consider what preparations would be necessary for dying in her own home. Despite the best planning, she ultimately found the hospital a more hospitable place to die. In the hospital, she felt safe. In the hospital, she would not suffocate. In the hospital, she was not alone.

For many years, my bias was no different than that of most people—the hospital is no place to die. I rarely witnessed patients dying well in acute-care institutions, and I believed that an art of dying could best be achieved *outside* such sterile environments.

However, as I have walked the final road with countless patients, I have gradually experienced more occasions when it just made sense to die in the hospital. Sometimes the problem is due to infrastructure: the house has too many stairs or the rooms are too small to accommodate needed medical equipment. Sometimes patients die in the hospital because their family dynamics prohibit dying well at home or because their communities cannot provide sufficient around-the-clock care. Sometimes patients are just too close to death to make it home.

Despite this, there exist many sound reasons to avoid hospital dying, and the most compelling of them have to do with the rescue fantasy. Doctors are hardwired to free patients from the grip of death, and patients are hardwired to seek safety. Procedures beget procedures, however, and these can provoke new kinds of suffering.

There are adverse events and unexpected complications. Medical equipment creates a barrier to physical touch. Some hospitals restrict the number of visitors and hours for visiting. Family members cannot necessarily sleep at the hospital. The hospital might be noisy. The patient may have a troublesome roommate. To top it off, the hospital provides extraordinarily expensive lodging for the dying—one night in intensive care can easily exceed $10,000. None of this sounds like the art of dying.

Although it is reasonable, then, to leave open the possibility of dying well in a hospital, it is also prudent to strategize about how to avoid it. When renowned violist and conductor Jesse Levine was diagnosed in 2008 with pancreatic cancer, he and his wife, Jill Pellett Levine, knew that the odds weren't in their favor. "One of the first conversations we had," Jill told me, "was about how to make it work for him to die at home." If he could die safely and comfortably, Jesse would die at home.

Levine was born in the Bronx in 1940, into a family of first- and second-generation Jewish Polish immigrants. His father, David, played the cello, and Jesse excelled at viola from an early age. He studied viola at Mannes College of the Arts and conducting with Igor Markevitch in Monaco. He was principal violist of multiple symphony orchestras around the United States, and he conducted several others. He filled a dual role of conductor and instructor to three youth orchestras in Spain. He loved to teach, and he was professor of viola and chamber music at the Yale School of Music for twenty-five years.

Despite an interest in dying at home, Jesse was not at all eager to die. In fact, as his finitude loomed, Jesse devoted himself all the more fully to his music. He continued to teach on Yale's campus until his strength failed, at which point the dean of the School of Music—himself highly supportive of Levine—arranged to send viola students out to Jesse's house by taxi.

Several weeks before he died, Jesse taught a master class from the hospital bed in his living room. He recognized that this would be the last opportunity to gather his students together, and in true *ars moriendi* fashion he used the occasion to exhort them:

> Being a musician, being your teacher, being at Yale, assisting in your growth has given me the greatest joy possible. Go and grow in your careers. Be generous, as you are, assisting each other whenever possible, unselfishly. We don't know what life may bring at any moment so support, support, support. I love each of you as if you were my own because music has brought us together.

With these words, he taught his last class.

Jesse had no illusion that his cancer would be cured, but he nevertheless insisted on receiving intravenous nourishment, known as total parenteral nutrition, or TPN. Typically TPN runs from a bag on an IV pole through tubing that traverses a flow-regulating pump before entering a large vein. Since Jesse was unable to eat enough by mouth to meet the demands of his cancer-ravaged body, he concluded that TPN would buy him some time. It probably did.

A few weeks before he died, the hospice nurse taught Jill how to disconnect the TPN so that Jesse could conduct for the last time. He had directed the New Britain Symphony Orchestra for several years by that point, and only death itself could keep him from a final performance. Jill felt less confident. "He looked like a ghost, he was so pale," she recalled. Jesse had hardly been out of bed in recent weeks, and his wife discreetly asked an orchestra member to support him onstage if he stumbled.

She needn't have worried. Decades of practice propelled the ailing conductor onward, and he led his musicians to a glorious finish. The maestro would not be thwarted.

As Levine engaged in the art of dying, his family and community accompanied him. Jill considered her role "an honor and privilege." She determined to support Jesse's flourishing as musician, teacher, father, and spouse—even as he lay dying. When he could no longer speak for himself, she spoke on his behalf, ensuring that all decisions about his medical care would uphold his dignity and humanity. Ultimately, he died at home as he had hoped—in the arms of his wife and sons.

Levine's example of an *ars moriendi* reminds us that the art of dying is wrapped up in the art of living. Stories like his should prompt us to prepare even now for death. When death threatens, we must keep our wits about us, guard against the allure of the hospital, and not rely on technology to absolve us of our fear of death.

None of this is easy. Discerning when a person actually stands to benefit from the hospital's offerings requires a reckoning with reality and frank conversations with medical professionals. Figuring out how to die at home requires planning—not just to acquire durable medical equipment such as a hospital bed, but also to organize family members and friends to work shifts. Most important, it requires the wisdom to discern when enough is enough and the will to shift attention from cure to care.

All of this becomes more complicated, however, when we fail to address the fear of death. To that subject we now turn.

CHAPTER FIVE

FEAR

No recent account of the fear of death surpasses that of the twentieth-century outbreak of plague in Oran, Algeria, as described in Albert Camus's novel *The Plague*. The Moors founded Oran on the Mediterranean coast around 900, but the Spanish, Ottomans, and French occupied it over the next thousand years. In Camus's telling, when the rats arrived in the 1940s—carrying the same plague that had infested Boccaccio's Florence some six hundred years earlier—the French had been living there for more than a century. And although they were once well versed in the *ars moriendi*, they had mostly forgotten its instruction. They avoided discussion of death and generally shunned the sick.

The rats provided the first clue that something was amiss. The day the plague surfaced, dead rats appeared everywhere— on sidewalks, in alleys, even in immaculately maintained apartment buildings. Within forty-eight hours, the garbage bins in front of each house were loaded with dead rodents. They were removed from factories in crates. On day three, city officials began transporting the carcasses by van to the town incinerator. One news source suggested that more than eight thousand rats had been burned in a single day.

Just when the quantity of rodent corpses threatened to overwhelm even the most stoic of citizens, officials announced that the sanitary service had collected far fewer rats. A mere twelve days had passed since the first had been discovered, and the inhabitants of Oran breathed a collective sigh of relief. They had not understood what had caused the blight, but they were glad it was nearly over.

Then a new calamity struck. People themselves started falling ill: they had fever, delirium, massively enlarging lymph nodes in the armpits and groin, and internal pains. For some, it became hard to breathe, and they started coughing up blood. If the rats were any sign of what was to come, this did not bode well. A thick fog of fear enveloped the coastal town.

Before the rats, the French residents of Oran had been comfortable in their ambivalence toward death. Even the historians among them were largely ignorant of the bubonic plague. They had never learned of the sixth-century Plague of Justinian in Constantinople, which the historian Procopius said had taken ten thousand lives in one day. Nor did they recall western Europe's fourteenth-century pandemic, which gave rise to the *ars moriendi*. Some might have heard of the more recent nineteenth-century outbreak in China's Yunan Province, where forty thousand rats died of plague before the first human became sick. The desire to avoid thoughts of mortality was stronger than the wish to recall human tragedy.

Even when their fellow citizens started dropping by a dozen a day, they preferred not to think of their finitude. The city was under quarantine, travel and sea bathing were forbidden, yet they carried on, as much as possible, in their normal routines. They hoped that the plague would end soon and that their families would be safe. Plague disrupted life in small ways, but it did not instill fear.

At the end of the first month of the plague, news sources began to advertise a special sermon to be preached by the local Jesuit priest, Father Paneloux. This sermon served to rouse the people of Oran from their existential slumber. Paneloux was known for his oratorical skills and dramatic flair. These he employed without hesitation. Camus recounts that Paneloux warned the townspeople that their proud hearts were responsible for the scourge; if they would humble themselves, God might remove the plague. It was hellfire and brimstone at its most passionate.

Perhaps the priest's sermon was to blame for stoking the people's fear, or perhaps not. Accounts vary. Suffice it to say that a widespread panic seized the town that same Sunday. By confronting the people with their mortality, the priest seemed to have led them to comprehend the significance of the plague for the first time.

The town of Oran sits nestled along the Mediterranean Sea, just east of the Straits of Gibraltar. Winters are mild and snowless, summers scorching. The week following the priest's call to repentance, temperatures shot up. So did the number of plague victims. The town's newly minted paper, *The Plague Chronicle*, stopped reporting weekly totals and began announcing them daily: 92, 107, 130. The heat sweltered, and fear swelled.

The townspeople responded in precisely the same manner as the fourteenth-century Florentines. Many shut themselves up inside their houses, drawing blinds and locking doors. Others spent their money lavishly. A visitor to Oran who later succumbed to plague recorded in his journal: "Daily, round about eleven, you see a sort of dress parade of youths and girls, who make you realize the frantic desire for life that thrives in the heart of every great calamity." Others restlessly took to the streets, provoking violent outbursts without apparent cause. Still others attempted to escape through the guarded city gates.

In that explosive mixture of heat and horror, lawlessness abounded. Trapped and desperate as the townsfolk were, the police force had no choice but to reorganize itself into a system of mounted patrols to rein in the frenzy. City officials began talking of conscripting healthy men into a sort of army that might take control of the plague by aggressive improvements in sanitation. But the very thought of being forcibly sent into battle against death itself only heightened fears. The degree of dread stood in direct proportion to death's proximity.

Waging War on Death

Fortunately, these events did not actually take place. Camus's famous 1947 work *The Plague* (*La Peste*) is fiction. Although not unheard of in Algeria at the time, plague cases were sporadic, not epidemic. Some believe Camus based his novel on a cholera outbreak in Oran almost a century earlier. Others think the story serves as a metaphor for French resistance to the Nazi occupation of France. Regardless of Camus's true intent, *La Peste* paints a vivid portrait of how disease can drive people from disengaged complacency about their finitude to a full-throttled fear of death—a fear that triggers them to attempt to take control of death by either waging war or escaping.

In the hospital today, descriptions of illness and disease are filled with the language of warfare. His grandfather is *battling* pneumonia. My friend is a cancer *survivor*. I'm going to *beat* this infection. She's a *fighter*; she's going to *kick* this disease. And so forth. We march forward, as determined as military generals, reminding our loved ones and ourselves that there is no reason to fear the enemy. We have the strongest health-care system of all time; no disease can conquer us.

In her 1978 book *Illness as Metaphor*, the literary giant Susan Sontag explains how the military metaphor was popularized in the 1880s, when bacteria were identified as "agents of
disease." Eventually, the language was appropriated for cancer.
In particular, Sontag writes: "Bacteria were said to 'invade' or
'infiltrate.' But talk of siege and war to describe disease now
has, with cancer, a striking literalness and authority. . . . [Can-
cer] itself is conceived as the enemy on which society wages
war." And to wage war, Sontag says, is to incite to violence,
which is precisely what the medical profession does. Doctors
commit acts of violence against cancer cells.

Sontag does not write about illness, cancer, and medicine
in the abstract. She knew them intimately. She was diagnosed
with stage IV breast cancer in 1975, uterine cancer in 1998,
and leukemia, a blood cancer, in 2004. She survived the first
despite the odds, at which point she wrote *Illness as Metaphor*.
She also beat uterine cancer, but leukemia would ultimately
defeat her.

Sontag was so terrified of death that she could not speak of
it. She could not bear the thought of her own death. Her son,
David Rieff, a writer in his own right, said, "in her eyes, mortality seemed as unjust as murder." She gravitated toward the
work of writers and artists who shared this fear, united with
them by a common inability to reconcile with human finitude. Sontag was not naive, of course. She could write about
death with unusual eloquence. And she fully understood that
one day she herself would die. But she just could not bring
herself to say it.

Despite Sontag's fear—or perhaps as a manifestation of it—
she was obsessed with death. She visited cemeteries—those in
Boston, Havana, Buenos Aires, London, and Montparnasse
were among her favorites. She even kept a human skull on her
worktable—a true memento mori. The fact that she refused
to resign herself to death "gave her the resolve," according to
her son, "to undergo any treatment, no matter how brutal, no
matter how slim her chances." The threat of death required of
Sontag's team a tactical response.

Sontag took control and went to war on her leukemia, encouraging her doctors to commit acts of extraordinary violence against the cancer that infiltrated her blood. Her only
chance at survival was a bone-marrow transplant, which, at
her age, was destined to fail. Her doctors told her that even if
she survived the transplant, her quality of life would be hor-
rendous. But this was a fight to the death against death itself,
and Sontag was ready for battle.

Rieff believes that his mother's desire to live was much
stronger than any other reality—even stronger than her fear
of death. Perhaps he is right. I cannot challenge the assessment
of a son who knew his mother so well. But when many of my
own patients, against insurmountable odds and innumerable
warnings, have committed themselves to experimental treatments that were bound to fail and destroy the quality of their
lives, the fear of death has seemed to be the driver—not the
desire to live. Perhaps when pushed to extremes, fear of death
and desire to live can best be understood as two sides of the
same coin.

Fear as Anger

A doctor-in-training asked me once how I make sense of those who are angry at the prospect of dying. She had lost her own mother to cancer, and she recounted that her mother had not been afraid to die; she had simply been incensed by the thought of death. Anger had motivated her to endure, as with Sontag, countless investigational treatments in the hope of living another day.

It is difficult to distinguish an all-consuming desire to live from a fear of death that compels one to fight. It is also difficult to distinguish fear of death from anger at the prospect of an untimely death. I have no doubt that the young doctor's mother was angry at the injustice of a disease that sought to pry her prematurely from the company of her family. But I do wonder whether fear didn't play a role. Fear famously masquerades as anger.

Most people fear death to some degree, even those who are certain that they have "made their peace." We naturally dread the perilous unknown. But not all fear compels a person to submit to torturous procedures that are unlikely to help. Given the choice between great suffering (with a slim chance at delaying death) and being made comfortable in their dying, some choose the latter. But not everyone.

Almost everything went wrong with Sontag's bone-marrow transplant. Rieff recalls sitting at his mother's hospital bedside in Seattle the day her doctors informed her that the transplant had failed and that her leukemia was taking over. She was too weak to roll over in bed without assistance, and a constant infusion of chemicals did nothing to help her condition. Sontag did not take the news well. According to Rieff, "She screamed out in surprise and terror. 'But this means I'm dying,' she kept saying, flailing her emaciated, abraded arms and pounding the mattress." She pleaded for more experimental treatments.

By the time she died, she had sores and bruises from mouth to sole. Still, Rieff believes that even if she could have fully understood from the beginning how much she would suffer, she would nevertheless have "rolled the dice and risked everything" for a little more time in this world. Raging against death, she urged her doctors to continue therapy even after she lost most of her lucidity, so great was her fear of her own extinction.

In the memoir Rieff wrote after his mother's death, he describes how he and all who were close to Sontag in her final months conspired to speak words of hope rather than truth. This was what she wanted, but such a conspiracy made it impossible to tell her that she was dying. They could not say goodbye properly or fully express their love for her—to do so would be to admit defeat. As a result, Rieff writes, "She who feared isolation and had the most terrible difficulties connecting with people had the loneliest of deaths."

The goal of controlling death compelled Susan Sontag and W. J. Turner's daughters to wage war. Still others plan an escape.

Escaping Death

We fear what we cannot control. In physiology—that branch of medical science that studies how living things function—we say that fear triggers a "fight or flight" response. When we feel threatened, we either fight back or run away. A cascade of nerve signals and hormones accelerates our heart and breathing, dilates our pupils to take in more light, and shuts down our digestion. When fighting for our lives, digestion-purposed, gut-bound blood is instead redirected to our muscles, enabling us to fight or run.

But how do we run from death?

Many people have argued that the practice of physician-assisted suicide, also known as aid in dying, offers a reasonable escape route from the dying process. Legal in a handful of US states, assisted suicide occurs when a medical doctor writes a lethal prescription and/or provides the necessary information for patients with terminal illnesses to end their lives themselves. It differs from euthanasia, which occurs when a doctor or nurse directly administers a deadly drug with the intention of hastening a patient's death. Euthanasia is illegal in most countries, including the United States, where it is considered murder.

Who chooses to escape dying through assisted suicide? Oregon provides us with more than two decades' worth of data on who requests lethal prescriptions and why. Most individuals are used to exercising a fair amount of control over their lives. They tend to be white, married or widowed, college-educated, and insured—a group that knows relative stability.

The reasons these patients give for seeking aid in dying highlight their desire to mitigate fear by controlling death through the "flight" element of "fight or flight." When asked about end-of-life concerns, about 90 percent say that they worry about losing their autonomy and being less able to participate in activities that make life enjoyable. In short, they fear losing control over their being and doing.

About three-quarters fear a loss of dignity. The State of Oregon does not define "dignity" for us, so we might adopt a standard *Oxford English Dictionary* definition: "the quality of being worthy or honorable." This in turn prompts the question: Why do the sick believe that dying strips them of their worth and honor? The very suggestion highlights how much we have lost the art of dying. If anything, the practices of the *ars moriendi* point to the deathbed as an opportunity for people to exercise dignity by dispensing words of hope and blessing to the family and friends who accompany them to their deaths. Such practices enhance, rather than diminish, dignity.

Perhaps when patients in Oregon say that they fear losing dignity, they are really describing the humiliation they feel when others have to assist them with personal tasks such as toileting and bathing. Indeed, just under half of those requesting lethal prescriptions in Oregon acknowledge worrying about losing control of bodily functions and becoming a burden on family and friends. Only about a quarter fear the possibility of inadequate pain control, which perhaps attests to the advances medicine has made with regard to pain relief.

Taken together, the data from Oregon paint a picture of patients from relatively secure backgrounds who seek to maintain that security in the face of an unpredictable dying process. For such patients, physician-assisted suicide offers the possibility of controlling death by choosing when and where and with whom they die.

All of us fear what we cannot control and aim to control what we fear. But does control of death truly mitigate fear? Or does it simply displace fear in the moment? How are the vast majority of dying patients—who desire neither futile medical treatments nor the premature termination of life—to deal with their fear?

Whether physician-assisted suicide is safe for vulnerable populations and whether medical doctors should be state-appointed agents of death are topics beyond the scope of this chapter. But what I wish to highlight is how assisted suicide provides an escape route for those who do not wish to fight death—but still want control.

Safe and Secure

Fear triggers a fight or flight response, and for the dying this can manifest as taking control by waging war on illness or by ending life prematurely. But what causes such fear? What is its source?

In the best of circumstances, children grow up healthy and happy. I say this knowing full well that I don't have to travel past hospital walls to know that many children grow up in poverty and violence, without access to caring families, nutritious food, good education, and health care. The worst is when children suffer both emotional *and* physical deprivation.

Those with physical deprivation but supportive communities can overcome adversity and thrive. Other children, like the young Susan Sontag, grow up in financial abundance but experience psychological abandonment. Sontag's father, a wealthy traveling furrier, died when she was five. Her emotionally distant mother remarried, and the new husband did not adopt Sontag and her sister. Feeling rejected and unloved, Sontag vowed to resist all defeat.

Regardless of our formative experiences, most of us give little thought to the various categories of safety for which we strive. We could probably agree that we desire physical safety—good health and freedom from physical harm. We seek a safe world, a hospitable world, a world that nurtures us through the air we breathe, the food we eat, the soil that yields our food. The beauty of nature adds richness to our lives. We invest in relationships, nourishment, and possessions to reinforce our sense of security.

But we also desire a sort of existential or ideological safety. By *ideology*, I mean a person's guiding philosophy of life, which may be religious in nature but is certainly not limited to religion. We reinforce our ideological security by associating with the like-minded: the similarly educated, politically persuaded, and socioeconomically classed. Or, as in Sontag's case, our existential safety is made real by our resistance to extinction.

I once had a patient whose wife told him that he should get a doctor when he turned sixty. So he came to see me. He was healthy, wealthy, and employed in a high-powered job. He boasted that he had not been to the doctor in decades. The small packet of records he brought to his new-patient visit, however, revealed several alarming health problems that he had managed to ignore.

I combed through his health history in detail, attending carefully to the red flags and formulating with him a plan for addressing each one. He seemed agreeable to it all, but when I suggested he schedule another appointment to follow up on the tests, he bolted for the door, bellowing, "I haven't been sick in twenty-five years, and I'm not going to start going to doctors now!" I never saw him again.

Only in retrospect did I realize how tightly he clung to the illusion that he had successfully evaded weakness. Like Sontag, he had constructed for himself a framework for physical and ideological safety that promised coherence for his life. And in that framework health problems had no place.

Unsafe and Afraid

When the natural world threatens, we take refuge in homes and cities. But when sickness threatens, we become homeless. Our own bodies evict us as if we were no longer welcome.

Our frames fail, our minds grow dim. Our stamina falters, and our work suffers. This, in turn, threatens our carefully constructed fortresses of security. As our physical space closes in, we stop being able to appreciate the beauty of the world. The poet Christian Wiman, himself a cancer survivor (to indulge Sontag's metaphor), says that pain "islands you." He writes: "You sit there in your little skeletal constriction of self—of disappearing self—watching everyone you love, however steadfastly they may remain by your side, drift farther and farther away."

Sickness makes our bodies inhospitable. But it also estranges us from our ideological framework. It is no longer enough to work hard. Ambition seems foolhardy, and prestigious careers offer false salvation. Stripped of our illusions, we find ourselves existentially isolated in our brokenness—perplexed in body and spirit.

The island of illness is much bigger than a basic realization of human finitude. "Let me tell you," Wiman asserts, "it is qualitatively different when death leans over to sniff you, when massive unmetaphorical pain goes crawling through your bones, when fear—goddamn fear, you can't get rid of it—ices your spine." Illness coalesces into incoherence. We find ourselves asking: *What did I do to deserve this? How could this happen to me?*

The threat of death robs us of physical and ideological safety and stokes our fear. The writer Simone Weil—whom Sontag once described as "one of the most uncompromising and troubling witnesses to the modern travail of the spirit"—

labeled this sort of total suffering *affliction*. Like Sontag and Wiman, Weil suffered from years of sickness. She betrays her deep intimacy with it in her writing:

> Affliction is anonymous before all things; it deprives its victims of their personality and makes them into things. It is indifferent; and it is the coldness of this indifference—a metallic coldness—that freezes all those it touches right to the depths of their souls. They will never find warmth again.

Sickness shows no restraint in its aptitude for uprooting lives and inculcating fear.

Sometimes the counsel of doctor, priest, or lover mitigates our dread. We find solace in the knowledge that the medication has no side effect, that the surgery has no downside, or that the doctor's prognosis was off by years. But then the disease resurfaces, and fear surges over us, overwhelms us, like a rising tide in the midst of a torrential downpour. Tossed overboard, we flail in cold dark waters.

Our well-intentioned fellow passengers try to rescue us. They pull us from the choppy waters, dress our wounds, and wrap us in warmth. Our fears recede, but only fleetingly. The storm of human finitude gathers new momentum. We are cast once again into the frigid sea ruled by a wild and incessant tempest. Fighting to keep our heads above the surface, we determine to take matters into our own hands. This is, after all, a matter of life and death. There is no placating this fear. The pacifying whispers of doctor, priest, or lover are swept away by the rising waters.

Dying into Life

The original *ars moriendi* offered a consolation for each of the five temptations faced by the dying: faith for the faithless; hope for the despairing; patience for the impatient; humility for the proud; and a relinquishing of earthly goods for the covetous. Despite their proximity to death, however, authors of the fifteenth-century art of dying failed to include fear as a central concern. How could this be?

Today fear of death is taken for granted. Dozens of my patients spring to mind—some broach the subject almost as a confession, while others, like Susan Sontag, refuse even to speak of it. Did fifteenth-century Europe not fear death in the same way?

Of course it did. Fear of death, which combines fear of the unknown with dread of extinction, doubtless dates back to the origins of humanity. But the degree to which early modern Europeans believed that they could *control* death pales in comparison to what we believe today. And since they knew well that there was very little to be done to thwart or delay death, they focused less on fear than on other aspects critical to dying, like despair or disbelief. In other words, if dying is inevitable—which they believed to be the case more truly than we do—one might as well strive to die well.

It is worth noting at this point that over the years there have been social authorities—particularly religious authorities in the *ars moriendi* tradition—who have suggested that those who fear death have not truly submitted themselves to God. On this point, the *ars moriendi* gets it wrong. Who wouldn't feel some reservation about a heretofore unexperienced life-altering event? Such teaching causes people to hide their fear of death and live poorly rather than to walk courageously toward it and die well.

We have seen already that breaches of safety prompt us to fear and that fear drives us to attempt to control what causes the dread. With regard to death, we attempt to mitigate our fear by waging war against it or by running from it through its intentional hastening. But both attempts ultimately sidestep the issue at hand. Sontag's story illustrates starkly how the struggle against death did nothing to address her fear. And physician-assisted suicide merely extinguishes fear by extinguishing the person who fears.

Some people think that by simply *accepting* death, a notion popularized by Elisabeth Kübler-Ross in her "five stages of grief," we will overcome such fear. But there are two problems with this. The first is that not everyone sails smoothly along Kübler-Ross's course: from denial to anger to bargaining to depression to acceptance. People rarely die algorithmically. And second, fear does not dissipate just because a person perfectly follows that path. There is no quick fix for the anxiety of death.

Those who have read this far will be disappointed that I prescribe no magic pill or incantation to conquer fear of death. But lessons from the stories of Susan Sontag and Camus's *Plague* are worth heeding. Sontag, who refused to discuss death, ultimately died in a sort of existential isolation. Camus's heroes, in contrast, walked straight into the plague, cared for the sick, eradicated rats, and improved sanitation. This was not glorious work—it was *moral* work—and it was necessary for the community, permitting those who participated to engage their fears of death while engaging with one another. "What accounts for the extraordinary appeal of [Camus's] work," Sontag once wrote, "is beauty of another order, moral beauty."

An intellectual titan, Sontag wrote admiringly of both Simone Weil and Albert Camus, two writers whose philosophical intuitions could not have been more opposed. She would doubtless have been similarly impressed by Christian Wiman, who has rapidly distinguished himself as one of the twenty-first century's most articulate poets.

Wiman tells the story of sitting with his grandmother as she died in the hospital. She seemed distressed, and so he asked her a series of questions to elicit the cause:

> Finally I asked—I did not want to—if she was scared and her eyes widened even farther and she began to shake terribly as she nodded yes and tried to form words around her breathing tube: yes, yes, yes. I suppose I don't know definitively whether she was afraid of dying or of further pain—she had been through so much by that time—but all my instincts argue for the former.

Wiman believes that his grandmother's fear of death is no indication that she died poorly. Instead, Wiman quotes the last words of poet Gerard Manley Hopkins, who died of typhoid in his forties. Hopkins said, "I am so happy. I am so happy. I loved my life." Wiman writes:

> How desperately we, the living, want to believe in this possibility: that death could be filled with promise, that the pain of leaving and separation could be, if not a foretaste of joy, then at least not meaningless. Forget religion. Even atheists want to die well, or want those they love to die well, which has to mean more than simply a quiet resignation to complete annihilation. . . . No, to die well, even for the religious, is to accept not only our own terror and sadness but the terrible holes we leave in the lives of others; at the same time, to die well, even for the atheist, is to believe that there is some way of dying into life rather than simply away from it, some form of survival that love makes possible.

This is Wiman's response to his grandmother's shaking fear of dying.

I am quite convinced that Wiman does not intend the dying to *accept* terror and sadness as if accepting them were some sort of task to be accomplished, a prescription to die well. Rather, he is nudging us toward moral work, toward Sontag's moral beauty. Wiman pushes us to walk courageously—with those we love—toward the terror and sadness, toward the holes we will inflict.

Will it all make sense? No. Will questions linger? Yes. Will we go to bed at night sad, confused, and angry? Very likely. But Wiman's counsel is to die *into* life rather than away from it. And the challenge for all of us is to figure out just what that means.

CHAPTER SIX

BODY

In July 1518, a different sort of plague struck western Europe. In the city of Strasbourg, in what is modern-day France, a certain Mrs. Troffea walked outside and started to dance. If she danced to music, no one heard it. Troffea twirled and leaped all day and into the night, at which point she collapsed from exhaustion. For a few hours she slept deeply. Upon awakening, she resumed her dance. Her perplexed husband gazed on, unable to reason with her.

By the third day of nearly incessant dancing, Troffea's feet were bloodied and bruised. Still she danced. A crowd of assorted onlookers had gathered to observe her mysterious, unremitting movements. Oblivious, she danced on. They discussed among themselves whether she was plagued by angels or demons. Deciding against the latter, they packed her into a wagon and transported her to a holy shrine up in the Vosges Mountains to commune with the divine.

The situation worsened. Within days, nearly thirty towns-people had taken to the streets similarly compelled to dance. As with Troffea, there seemed to be no stopping them. They perspired profusely, leaped and contorted unwittingly, as if driven by something stronger than individual will. If they rested at all, the respite was brief. They seldom ate or drank. Others joined the madness. Within about a week, more than a hundred people were dancing in the streets of Strasbourg.

At first the authorities thought that the best cure was to let the afflicted dance it out. They reserved guildhalls and hired professional musicians and dancers to keep the people on their feet. But frenzy begat frenzy, and Strasbourg officials quickly determined that encouraging the riotous behavior led to disas-trous consequences. By the end of a month, the dancing mania had struck four hundred people. Many succumbed to dehy-dration, heart attacks, strokes, and exhaustion. Their bodies broke.

The Dancing Plague

Numerous contemporaries documented the bizarre event—city officials, scholars, merchants, clergy, and even an archi-tect. Some described Strasbourg's 1518 dancing plague in real time. Others wrote about it a decade or two later. As printing presses spread their accounts, everyone hoped that the mystery would one day be solved.

Strasbourg's epidemic may be the world's best-documented outbreak of the dancing plague, but it is not the only one. Such manic dancing dates back as far as the seventh century, and there are accounts of outbreaks in German and Welsh towns in 1017 and 1188, respectively. German chronicles record episodes in 1247 and 1278. The largest epidemic spread along the Rhine River in 1374. Several other western European episodes punctuated the subsequent two centuries.

Even today, no one really knows what triggered it, but two theories have emerged. The first is that the dancing plague was caused by ergot poisoning. Ergot comes from a fungus, *Claviceps purpurea*, which can grow on grains, especially rye, in damp climates after a cold winter. Although the temperatures in western Europe throughout the Middle Ages typically prevented the growth of large concentrations of *Claviceps*, damper and colder years caused the fungus to flourish. Farmers inadvertently ground ergot together with rye grains into toxic flour. Since rye bread was a dietary staple, entire communities could suffer.

Ergot is the same chemical from which the psychedelic drug LSD was isolated in 1938. It works by constricting small blood vessels in the arms, legs, and brain. Several days after consuming toxic rye bread, the "trip" begins: nausea, vomiting, diarrhea, and a sensation of bugs crawling on the skin. Muscles then begin to contract involuntarily and painfully.

Victims experience auditory and visual disturbances. Then the scourge typically takes one of two turns—it becomes gangrenous or convulsive.

The gangrenous form develops as the blood vessels in the arms and legs constrict, cutting off blood flow. The tissues of toes, fingers, hands, and feet die and auto-amputate. Constricted blood flow also means that the appendages do not bleed. The ears and nose are commonly affected, leading to extreme disfigurement.

But it is the convulsive form that many believe accounts for dancing-plague epidemics. Ergot restricts blood flow to the brain, causing muscle twitching and spasms, mania, mental confusion, hallucinations, and other forms of psychosis. If medical research on LSD from the 1960s is anything to go by, LSD use (and perhaps also ergot poisoning) can lead to "suggestibility," meaning that those intoxicated are more susceptible to influences than they would be normally—which is why hiring musicians to encourage the afflicted to "dance it out" made matters worse.

The historian John Waller offers the other leading explanation for the dancing plague. He understands epidemics of dancing to be responses to a combination of horrific circumstance, suggestibility, and profound religious belief. For example, the largest known outbreak of the dancing plague occurred in 1374, two decades after the bubonic plague. Waller posits that "psychic disintegration" induced trancelike states of hallucinogenic, manic dancing that were in turn invigorated by sensations of religious ecstasy.

The Cursed Bread

No one, of course, will ever be able to prove what precisely transpired on that Strasbourg street some five hundred years ago. Was Mrs. Troffea suffering from ergot poisoning? Or was she simply experiencing a psychological break exacerbated by superstition and hyperreligiosity? Although it is not inconceivable that the two theories could somehow converge, a twentieth-century episode in the small town of Pont-Saint-Esprit in southern France suggests that we should not dismiss fungus poisoning as the cause of the dancing plague.

On August 16, 1951, a large number of people ate bread from a single bakery. Within hours, they became agitated. They developed abdominal pain, nausea, vomiting, and diarrhea. Some described a choking sensation. Next, they felt gusts of warmth followed by waves of cold. They experienced intense sweating and drooling. Their hearts beat more slowly. Their hands and feet grew cold. After this they developed insomnia, which lasted for several days. They felt as if their insides were burning. They were giddy. They trembled.

Animals that ate the bread scraps also behaved erratically. Ducks marched erectly like penguins, flapped their wings, and died. A crazed dog bounded through the air, sprinted in circles, chewed rocks until its teeth disintegrated, and also died.

About twenty-five of the three hundred or so human cases progressed to the most severe form. Insomnia persisted, and the victims began to shake, twitch, and grow increasingly agitated. Some babbled and moved incessantly. They hallucinated, convinced they were confronting horrid animals and consuming fires. Then followed a dreamy delirium.

Within the month, several French medical doctors described the symptoms in the *British Medical Journal*. In the most severe cases:

> The delirium seemed to be systematized, with animal hallucinations and self-accusation, and it was sometimes mystical or macabre. In some cases terrifying visions were followed by fugues, and two patients even threw themselves out of windows. The delirium was of a confusional kind which could be interrupted for some moments by strong stimulation. Every attempt at restraint increased the agitation.

Four of the people among the twenty-five severest cases died. Their hearts gave out under the combination of insomnia and constant movement. One of the dead had gangrenous toes.

As the *New York Times* described it, the behavior of the afflicted went from bad to worse. Some became so crazy, they were locked up:

> A worker tried to drown himself because his belly was being eaten by snakes. A 60-year-old grandmother threw herself against the wall and broke three ribs. A man saw his heart escaping through his feet and beseeched a doctor to put it back in place. Many were taken to the local asylum in strait jackets.

The most credible explanation? Something in the bread baked on the night of August 15.

Altarpiece Therapy

For centuries, no one knew what caused the gangrene, convulsions, and LSD-like psychosis. They called it "St. Anthony's fire" after the third-century Christian monk whose relics reportedly healed a nobleman's son of the disease. "Fire" referred to the burning feeling that victims described in their guts, arms, and legs. Ergot as its causative agent was not discovered until the seventeenth century.

According to tradition, the nobleman, grateful for his son's healing, founded the Order of St. Anthony in 1095 in southwestern France. The order's mission was to care for those who suffered from St. Anthony's fire, among other illnesses such as the bubonic plague. It built hospitals throughout France, eventually expanding into Germany, Italy, and Spain. At its peak, the order boasted some 370 hospitals.

During the early stages of assembling this book, the painter Linnéa Spransy alerted me to a five-hundred-year-old masterpiece dedicated to victims of St. Anthony's fire. Spransy had been on a grand tour of European contemporary art, but had broken her modern stride to view the famous Isenheim Altarpiece painted by Matthias Grünewald. The multipaneled work was originally commissioned for the Antonite order in Isenheim, France, but is now housed in a convent turned museum in the medieval city of Colmar. The Isenheim Altarpiece is not an ordinary piece of religious art. It depicts the broken body of the crucified Christ as afflicted with St. Anthony's fire.

Altarpieces have been used for a thousand years to beautify churches and to tell stories. They are painted and sculpted works, typically placed in the very front of the church, for devotion and instruction. But the Isenheim Altarpiece had an additional function. The Antonites "prescribed" viewing of the altarpiece to those in their care who were suffering from St. Anthony's fire. The Antonites would distribute fresh bread and *saint vinage*, a drink of wine and healing plants into which they had dipped Anthony's relics. They would then lead the sick into the choir area of Isenheim church, where they could meditate on the cosuffering of Christ. The altarpiece assured the sick that Christ understood their pain.

I was intrigued that a painting of a plague-infested body of Christ could be used as art therapy, and I embarked on a mission to learn more. It turns out that Grünewald's altarpiece is a subject over which much ink has been spilled.

The American novelist Francine Prose described the Isenheim Altarpiece as "life-changing." She was astonished to find that "at some point in our history, a society thought that this was what art could do: that art might possibly accomplish something like a small miracle of comfort and consolation." The Austrian-born Jewish philosopher Martin Buber was so moved by his visit to the Isenheim Altarpiece that he penned his essay "The Altar" and dedicated it to the masterpiece. Grünewald's altarpiece also influenced the French artist Henri Matisse's vision for the chapel of Notre-Dame-du-Rosaire in Venice.

But it was an essay by the nineteenth-century French art critic Joris-Karl Huysmans that moved me to see the altarpiece for myself. Huysmans writes of Grünewald:

> There, in the old Unterlinden convent, he seizes on you the moment you go in and promptly strikes you dumb with the fearsome nightmare of a *Calvary*. It is as if a typhoon of art had been let loose and was sweeping you away, and you need a few minutes to recover from the impact, to surmount the impression of awful horror made by the huge crucified Christ dominating the nave of this museum.

Strikes you dumb? Typhoon of art? I determined to see it.

Pretzels and Magic

Colmar's promotional photographs typically show one of two kinds of scenes: nighttime shots of cheery Christmas markets tidily traced by strings of festive lights or summertime photographs of sixteenth-century wood-frame houses, with flowers spilling from planters, over narrow canals. I planned my trip over spring vacation, expecting sunny weather and the first flowers of spring.

It was late on a Saturday evening in mid-March when the train from Paris pulled slowly into the Colmar station. It was snowing. The handful of others who disembarked with me dissipated into the flake-speckled darkness. The streets were empty and quiet. Snow smothered every sound.

Observing no taxi, I ventured forth on foot, through several inches of snow, toward the city's center. The snow in my shoes and on my face failed to vex. Snow has always filled me with awe, especially at night when it first blankets the world in silence. "Behold the snowflake exquisite in form," writes the poet Rollo Russell. That tiny crystals can form such majestic lattices, completely transforming a landscape, demands reverence.

After a quarter hour of walking I arrived at the outskirts of the historic center. It felt like a theatrical set for a production of the Grimm brothers' fairy tales. Three- and four-story wood-frame buildings painted in yellows and oranges nestled together along winding pedestrian streets and footpaths. The shops were closed, but their lit windows displayed sumptuous chocolates, pretzels, breads, and dried fruit. Colmar could make the most ardent materialist believe in magic.

Next morning, the sky was gray, the ground slushy, and the falling snow reduced to a few flurries. By all appearances, Colmar had become more *real* and less *sur*real. But with images of the previous night imprinted on my mind, the fairy-tale spirit of the place hung about me like a cloak.

Hybrid Creature

I arrived at the Unterlinden Museum twenty minutes before opening. I had been told that the best time to view the Isenheim Altarpiece was first thing in the morning, before the tour groups arrived. I paced back and forth in front of the locked door, wondering if the altarpiece would be as "life-changing" for me as it had been for Prose or Buber or Matisse. I wondered if it would inspire my writing. I wondered why they couldn't open the door early, especially for me, just this once. . . .

My meditation was interrupted by the arrival of a remarkably well-behaved group of French kindergarteners. It was their annual school field trip to the art museum. They too were early. I eyed them with a mixture of admiration for their orderliness and despair that they would ruin my first encounter with the Isenheim Altarpiece. Thinking of my own children, I tried hard to cultivate a charitable posture.

The doors opened precisely at the advertised hour. I sneaked swiftly past the brightly booted brood and up to the ticket counter. In less than a minute, I was walking through the cloister of the old convent courtyard and into the space of the former chapel that housed the wonder.

And there he was. That anguished man on a cross, larger than life, bearing all the marks of ergotism. His skin was covered in sores from whipping and disease, his lips and toes tinted blue, his spindly fingers splayed open, the tips twisting around the nails in his hands. Borrowing from Abraham Heschel, this is Jürgen Moltmann's "pathetic" Christ—one with *pathos*, one who suffers.

In the panel to his left stands Anthony, who heals and protects from St. Anthony's fire. The panel to his right portrays Sebastian, patron saint of archers and bubonic-plague sufferers. The message of the composition goes beyond the familiar "Christ died for you." It tells viewers, "Christ suffers and dies right alongside you, victim of the plague, of St. Anthony's fire. His body is ruined like yours. He understands your pain. You are not alone."

The Isenheim Altarpiece is composed of a number of painted panels and sculptures that were opened and closed depending on holidays and the seasons of the liturgical year. Typically, viewers would have gazed upon the crucified Christ. But sometimes, patients and pilgrims sat before another panel, seldom opened, called "Saint Anthony Tormented by Demons." No amount of research had prepared me for this painting.

Legend has it that Anthony, who was born into a wealthy family, gave his riches to the poor in favor of a hermit's life. Aspiring to solitary communion with God, he moved to the desert. The stories suggest that on at least two occasions Anthony was assaulted by demons who sought to tempt him back to his former life of comfort and pleasure. He nearly died after the first attack, but a friend discovered his thrashed body and nursed him back to health. Anthony insisted on returning to the desert, where the demons again sought to destroy him. This is what Grünewald depicts in colors more vivid than any reproduction attests.

In Grünewald's painting, Anthony has been flung to the ground and a pack of hideous beasts attacks him from all sides. A fingerless appendage clutches Anthony by the hair. A stubby yellow claw—perhaps attached to a golden-winged arm and shark jaw with canine nose—steps on Anthony's chest. There are others: a ghoul with short spiked antlers eats Anthony's cloak, a dog's black snout with feathered mane hovers like an apparition, a green-winged bicorn beast prepares to pounce.

It is impossible to tell where one creature stops and another begins. Anthony is nearly overcome by an amalgam of claws, teeth, jaws, feathers, and weapons clutched for slaughter. If the beasts are victorious, Anthony will fail to become Anthony the Great, patron saint of the suffering sick.

The eye is first drawn to the demons, and second to Anthony himself, who raises his arm to shield his face. But there is another being in the lower left corner, neither vicious beast nor truly human. He sits back on his haunches, grimacing face cast upward, legs spread wide, bloated belly pushing against the surrounding darkness. His skin is littered with the haloed lesions of St. Anthony's fire. His feet are webbed, his left arm a gangrenous stump. As Huysmans puts it:

> Whatever it may be, one thing is certain: no painter has ever gone so far in the representation of putrefaction, nor does any medical textbook contain a more frightening illustration of skin disease. This bloated body, moulded in greasy white soap mottled with blue, and mamillated with boils and carbuncles, is the hosanna of gangrene, the song of triumph of decay!

This pathetic hybrid personifies bodily suffering. Disease disfigures as it transforms.

The decay of our physical bodies, as Huysmans says, ultimately does triumph. Whether bubonic or dancing plague, heart attack or stroke, malignancy or senility, all of us experience little deaths in our bodies as we march slowly toward our corporeal end. Finitude on a small scale—the rickety knee, the bifocals—ought to stir in us a need to prepare for that final finitude.

Our journeys of bodily decline will doubtless vary. Some of us will develop cancer, undergo grueling treatments, and enter a period of remission—only to be devastated years later by its vengeful return. Others will develop slowly progressing chronic diseases, such as diabetes or heart failure. As our health deteriorates, we will experience more frequent hospital tune-ups, until that last hospitalization.

Some of us will experience health "scares"—that curable cancer or that massive heart attack from which we recover. We vow to change our unhealthy habits and to see each day as a gift. But that encounter with mortality has shaken us. Others will live to a ripe old age, succumbing to the clouded confusion of dementia or to an acute illness like pneumonia, "the old man's friend." Regardless, our physical bodies are forever altered by our confrontations with illness.

I care for an elderly patient who has been struggling with a chronic debilitating disease for most of his adult life. But that chronic disease is the least of his worries. What really makes him feel like a "little old man" is his arthritis. Now in his late seventies, the nagging pain keeps him from exercising, working in the garden, or playing bridge. Recently he told me that he is ready to give up.

The disfiguration caused by disease alienates us from ourselves and from our communities. For some, it feels as though the cosmos itself has cursed us and left us for dead. In the lower right corner of Grünewald's painting, directly across from the miserable hybrid creature, a piece of parchment is tacked to a tree stump. On it are written the words Anthony purportedly uttered when finally liberated from the demons: *Ubi eras, Ihesu bone, ubi eras, quare non affuisti ut sanares vulnera mea?* "Where were you, O good Jesus, where were you? Why did you not come sooner to help me and heal my wounds?"

This is the same question that a Jewish woman named Martha ostensibly asked Jesus when her brother Lazarus died. According to the story from the Gospel of John, Jesus receives word that his friend Lazarus is sick and plans to travel to see him. By the time Jesus arrives, Lazarus has been dead and buried for four days, and a group of Jewish mourners has gathered at the house to console the family.

Martha wants to know why Jesus did not come sooner to heal her brother. He indirectly replies that her brother will rise again. Martha responds by appealing to a common first-century Jewish belief: "I know that he will rise again in the resurrection on the last day." Jesus, also Jewish, insists that he is not talking about the eventual bodily resurrection of the dead. Instead, he tells Martha that *he* is the resurrection and the life: "Those who believe in me, even though they die, will live." If

this riddle leaves Martha perplexed, she is even more astonished when Jesus summons the dead man out of the tomb and
back to life.

Although modern medicine works hard to resuscitate dead
bodies, I have never witnessed the successful resuscitation of
a four-day-old corpse. My guess is that most of us relate more
to the question *Why did you not come sooner to help me and
heal my wounds?* than to miraculous resurrection. Our failing
bodies cause us grief. No one is exempt.

Even Christ on the cross felt the sting of his wounds. "My
God, my God, why have you forsaken me?" Illness drives our
feelings of abandonment, giving rise to deep, visceral cries.
We direct our pleas toward God, toward our doctors, or toward the universe itself. *Why me? Why this? Who will heal my
wounds?*

Forsaken

In reflecting on this sense of total abandonment, the philosopher John Hare once asked, "But how could Jesus be forsaken
by his Father?" Hare answered his own question by relating
Christ's experience of forsakenness to human experiences of
physical suffering:

> Imagine yourself in hospital with chest pains, and they poke
> needles into you in many different parts of your body at
> many hours of the day and night; they deprive you of food

and water; all around you are the sounds of pain and distress; you are made entirely passive, with all your agency taken away, and there is ever-present the thought of death; and your medical persecutors do not seem to know what they are doing: they know not what they do.

The experience of illness produces the experience of forsakenness, of abandonment. Our families and friends, even our doctors, have no idea what to do with us. So they leave us alone with our wounds and our bloated bellies, and there we sit in misery, the demons of death thrashing about us.

If the Isenheim Altarpiece changed my life in one way, it was through its illustrations of failing bodies—open sores, blue lips, twisted appendages, gangrenous stumps. It was through its depiction of the horror that sickness and death inflict on the individual and the community. As a medical doctor, I have too often witnessed the disfiguring effects of disease. But such effects are not so fixed and frozen in time as they are in a painting. One cannot help being disturbed by the anguished face that persists in painted form, unable to experience relief. The viewer's ultimate response is to look aside, to forsake the one who suffers.

At the end of the day, I left the Unterlinden Museum. I walked away from the images of suffering. And at the end of each day, I go home from work. Sometimes I walk away from the images of my suffering patients. But not always. Sometimes I take their suffering home with me, though they do not know it. And only occasionally can I shut them out of my mind entirely. Although the healthy may be able to ignore the physical suffering around them, those who suffer from illness can never shut out their own misery of body.

It might seem odd to include in a book on the art of dying a chapter that serves as a meditation on the decay of the body. Why focus on the grit? The truth of the matter is that this chapter is not necessary for the sick and hurting. They already know anguish far too well. But the healthy remainder of the population can use a reminder of bodily finitude—their own and that of others. This chapter is intended to open our eyes to the physical suffering around us, to inspire us not only to expect it, but also to contemplate how we might accompany the frail and broken among us.

Some religious traditions make a point of encouraging re-flection on human brokenness. Ash Wednesday—known best for black smudges on the foreheads of the faithful—is one such occasion. Ash Wednesday marks the beginning of Lent, a forty-day season during which Christians prepare themselves for Easter through prayer, repentance, and fasting. Some churches hold special services for the "imposition of ashes" on the face—an outward sign of an inward process.

I was working on this chapter when Ash Wednesday rolled around, and I decided to attend the service at my Episcopal church. Night had fallen. Entering the church a few minutes late, I couldn't help but notice that a somber, serious tone hung in the air. Every reading, every recitation seemed to point toward death. Death to self. Death of sin. Human mor-tality. Christ himself would have to die before Easter could come. His admirers would have to die to self before they could follow him.

After a brief preamble describing the development of the tradition of ashes, the priest cut to the chase. "Almighty God, you have created us out of the dust of the earth: Grant that these ashes may be to us a sign of our mortality and penitence." After the "Amen," I joined my fellow congregants in line to receive the ashes.

It had been some years since I had attended this service, and as I stepped forward to face the priest, I closed my eyes. I wasn't sure if I was supposed to close my eyes, but it seemed right. With his thumb, the priest signed a cross of gritty ashes on my forehead while declaring, "Remember that you are dust, and to dust you shall return." I noticed how the ash between his thumb and my forehead crunched some as he applied it—the further disintegration of previously charred matter. To dust it all returns.

Dismembered and Consumed

The Isenheim Altarpiece was commissioned for a monastic order that cared for victims of the dancing plague and the bubonic plague. Its function was therapeutic—consoling, comforting, offering solidarity. The patients who sat in its presence ate bread and drank *saint vinage* while contemplating ancient stories of suffering and redemption. There was a certain wholeness about the experience, a quietude, a reflection on corporeal finitude and its attendant spiritual preparation, a reverence for the mystery that is life and death.

Today, the altarpiece has been dismantled and dismembered, all of its panels and sculptures simultaneously on display for consumption by visitors in relative health. It is housed not in a hospital or church, but in the deconsecrated chapel of a former convent turned first-class museum. The sick no longer take refuge in its presence. If this masterpiece once belonged to the "art of dying" tradition, it no longer does. It is simply "art"—to be consumed.

In some ways, the bodies of patients share a similar fate. Today, doctors have dismantled and dismembered the bodies of patients, dividing their various organ systems among a host of specialists with relative health and privilege. Medical treatments occur in a sterile clinical context, devoid of the histories and stories that enrich our lives. Doctors and other health professionals focus on bodies and ignore spirits, and the broader public has acquiesced. Despite professed commitments to "holistic care," most of our treatments remain biological, chemical, and procedural—addressing what can be rationalized and measured and assessed. So many deaths—like that of Susan Sontag—are unartful, disenchanted.

Many will argue that the Isenheim Altarpiece belongs in a museum, guarded and protected and available to all who can pay. I probably agree. But one question remains. Can doctors care well for patients—and can we care well for one another—when we treat bodies as collections of organs rather than as human beings whose capacities and beliefs surpass the purely material? The answer, surely, is *no*. However we may think about our lives, there is something there that is more than what can be measured and assessed. There is more than the strictly material, which is why we next consider the spirit, a subject that physician-writers in recent years have largely left untouched.

CHAPTER SEVEN

SPIRIT

Late one night, the nurses paged me. My patient Edith Blatchley was being "noncooperative"—a medical euphemism for feisty, spirited, difficult. Ms. Blatchley was eighty-six. A former factory worker and the oldest child in a working-class family, she had never married because she didn't want to give up her job. She was fiercely independent and had lived on her own until she fractured her hip. Breaking a hip and losing her freedom frightened her, but what was really petrifying was the prospect of death: mortality after a hip fracture is high, and she had suffered every possible complication.

I found her with her hospital bedsheet clutched in her spidery fingers, pulled taut to her chin. Beneath the sheet, I could see the outline of her rigid wasted body. Her eyes were clenched shut, as if squeezing could banish the specter of death.

"Ms. Blatchley," I whispered, my hand on her shoulder. "It's Dr. Dugdale. Are you okay?"

Her eyes popped open, angry and frightened. "I'm dying," she seethed. "What happens when I die? I don't know what I believe."

I tried to ask questions, to get a sense of what prompted her outrage, but the various infections that plagued her body vied for her attention. Our conversation made little headway. She died before the week was over—another loss to the living.

Religion Nonsense

I live at the intersection of three institutions: university, medical center, and church. Many of my work colleagues bristle at the thought of religion—at least in its traditional forms. Yoga and mindfulness are fine, they might say, but dogma and theology? Not so much.

One day I surprised myself with my response to a fellow professor's off-the-cuff comment about "all that religion nonsense." I found myself saying, "Yes, but my job is to take care of sick and dying people. Almost everyone becomes religious when they're dying." Perhaps this is an overstatement—at least in a New England university town. But the fact remains: many people do become interested in larger existential questions as they confront death.

Take, for example, a long-standing patient of mine who came to my office for her annual exam. She seemed uncharacteristically flustered. Despite this, I chose to start our visit the way I usually do. "I know you're here for your regular checkup, but is there anything in particular you wanted to make sure we cover today?"

The words had hardly left my mouth when she blurted out, "I just had my seventieth birthday. *Seventy!* For the first time I realized that I am closer to death than not. And I have no idea what I believe. I mean, I was brought up Methodist, but I left the church years ago. Do I believe in life after death? I don't know!"

For her age, my patient was in impeccable health. But she had arrived at the psalmist's prescribed threshold, and "threescore years and ten" had catapulted her from complacency to soul searching. She spent the rest of her visit posing existential questions; the prospect of death had forced her to reflect on the meaning of life.

Religion Lite

Over the course of my experience as a physician, many patients have wanted to process questions of death, meaning, and purpose. Why am I here? What is this life for? What happens when I die? Such questions are accurately described as existential—they are after all questions about human *existence*. But for the majority of the world's population, for most Americans, and for many of my patients in the semi-secularized Northeast, these questions are religious.

Religions offer particular systems of thought that provide coherence and overarching narratives for human experience. Contrary to some popular thinking, faith is not defined as blind obedience. Rather, it is a commitment or relationship to a divine person or set of principles. Religion is a practice that makes sense of our particular slice of the world on the basis of shared commitments and practices.

Forty years ago, there was consensus among sociologists that the world was becoming less religious; modernization had led to secularization in western Europe, and the rest of the world was expected to follow. Although this hypothesis has been found false in the decades since, many coastal Americans (particularly white male Americans) are less interested in religion than were previous generations. But spirituality remains intriguing. The Pew Research Center—the nonpartisan American "fact tank" that studies public opinion on a wide variety of issues—summarized this point in an article titled: "Americans May Be Getting Less Religious, but Feelings of Spirituality Are on the Rise."

In my own work caring for dying patients, I have found that this sort of spirituality is at its core a "religion lite"—a low-calorie attempt to make sense of the world free from dogma and constraint. If generational caricatures have validity, then religion lite should appeal to our current generations.

The free-spirited, individualistic baby boomers are in positions of senior management, eager to be "nonauthoritarian" authorities who do not impose any principle too forcefully. Their children, the cynical yet pragmatic Generation Xers, who value a balance between work and life, are reaching mid-career. Gen Xers are trying to make sense of the world by acting more grown-up than their parents and providing more structure for their children than their parents provided for them.

Finally, we have the Millennials—the "least religious generation." Millennials are less likely to be religious or spiritual than the two generations before them. And although most still identify at least on paper with a particular religion, many are attracted to religion lite.

Existential Explanations

Despite generational shifts, existential questions somehow have a way of persisting. For my patients, existential anxiety rises to the surface when mortality looms large. Previous generations, as we have seen, relied on the *ars moriendi* to provide the language necessary for exploring such concerns. But the medieval art of dying no longer holds sway. In fact, the prevailing sentiment seems to be, according to British theologian N. T. Wright, that traditional beliefs, like those concerning judgment, hell, and resurrection, are actually "offensive to modern sensibilities." We have figured out other ways to talk about life after death.

Wright describes three main beliefs about life after death that compete with the religious orthodoxy of the Judeo-Christian

West. The first is the idea of "complete annihilation"—when the body is dead, it is done. The philosopher Shelly Kagan characterizes it best:

> There is no soul; we are just machines. Of course, we are not just any old machine; we are *amazing* machines. . . . And when the machine breaks, that's the end. . . . Ultimately, death is no more mysterious than the fact that your lamp or your computer can break or that any machine will eventually fail.

This is complete annihilation. There is nothing after death. The dead are simply broken machines that turn to dust.

The second is reincarnation, and there are several types. Some endorse a sort of reincarnation with loose ties to Hindu, Buddhist, New Age, or even Judeo-Christian ideas. Operative here is a literal cycle of death and rebirth; it is believed that creatures who have died are reborn on earth as different beings. Others endorse the idea of reincarnation for the purposes of psychoanalysis and self-improvement—"discovering aspects of your personality that come from who you were or what happened to you in a previous life." Still others believe that the dead are absorbed into the wind or the trees—language we often hear at funerals. "I know she is here with us," a mourner might say. "She lives on in our hearts."

One example of the last type of reincarnation blends nature religion with a lingering belief in a generic immortality. After Diana, Princess of Wales, died, Wright says that a message was found in London written as if in her own words: "I did not leave you at all. I am still with you. I am in the sun and in the wind. I am even in the rain. I did not die, I am with you all." Sentiments such as this can be part of good faith efforts to hold on to the recently deceased and to keep memories alive.

The third notion about life after death is tied to a belief in ghosts or spiritualistic contact with the dead. Ghost sightings and Ouija boards are among the most popular demonstrations of this belief. The American poet James Merrill, for instance, reported prior to his own death that he wrote his award-winning epic poem *The Changing Light at Sandover* based on two decades of messages dictated from otherworldly spirits during Ouija-board séances.

Whether it be complete annihilation, some version of rein-carnation, or a deliberate spiritualistic contact with the dead, Wright suggests that at some point most of us embrace one or another of these attitudes toward life after death. Perhaps he's right. Or maybe these categories are too simplistic to char-acterize all people who hold nontraditional Western views of life and death. But maybe some of us have never given it much thought.

Spiritual but Not Religious

One of the problems I often wrestle with as a doctor who in-teracts with patients in secular health-care settings is whether a nonspecific spirituality suffices to address the existential qualms of patients like Ms. Blatchley. Isn't a fuzzy answer to life's ultimate mysteries akin to wrapping gauze around a gangrenous leg? Others think that a nonspecific spirituality, if anything, should be able to satisfy general existential concerns.

Take the Canadian social worker and civil rights and environmental activist John Shields. His was a life of service, but as an ex-Catholic, he was also dedicated (in the words of his biographer) to "freedom—intellectual, spiritual, personal. He was always growing and exploring." In his last few months of life, he experimented with psychedelic drugs and took an online course on transcending transpersonal realms.

When he was dying of an incurable disease called amyloidosis, the *New York Times* reported that he chose to celebrate an Irish wake with friends and family prior to being euthanized. After the lethal injection, his body was laid in his garden for two days, because his wife believed that his spirit would stay with the body for a period before journeying on. Celebrated as a man who takes life and death on his own terms, he didn't "get religion" in the conventional sense of the term. Does that matter?

Many people—perhaps most—think not. Being spiritual but not religious (SBNR), they assert, should satisfy any spiritual hankerings. Religious studies professor Robert Fuller argues in his book *Spiritual but Not Religious* that conventional churchgoing is no longer an option for millions of Americans; therefore "unchurched" spiritual traditions provide the beliefs and practices that make it possible "to reject a purely materialistic view of life." Compared with their religious counterparts, Fuller says, unchurched spiritual seekers take greater interest in mysticism and the unorthodox. They tend to focus on inner sources of spirituality, and they are more willing to experiment with their beliefs and change them as needed.

Fuller is quick to note that SBNR individuals differ from the secular nonreligious on two main points—a distinction originally articulated by the psychologist William James. First, the SBNR remain convinced that the world is embedded in a spiritual universe. And second, they hold that the purpose of life is to find harmony with this spiritual realm. The secular nonreligious, by contrast, conceive of a strictly material universe devoid of a spiritual realm.

Many religious people, however, remain skeptical of the SBNR position. They maintain that only a carefully articulated religion—"a particular system of faith and worship" as the *Oxford English Dictionary* defines it—can fully aspire to satisfy a person's deepest existential struggles.

One such critic is Lillian Daniel, author of the book *When "Spiritual but Not Religious" Is Not Enough.* Daniel describes the SBNR worldview as a product of secular American consumer culture, far removed from community. Daniel's approach is tongue-in-cheek and likely off-putting to those who derive meaning from being SBNR. But the essence of her concern is that people who favor SBNR can believe what they want and practice when they want without having to commit to established creeds or traditions. They prefer, in essence, a choose-your-own-god adventure.

Since SBNR is not enough for Daniel, she proposes an antidote: commitment to a religious community. Hardly surprising coming from a church minister. However, she goes on to admit that there are many embarrassing reasons she would rather not be associated with the Christian church. Some of its members, as with society at large, are frankly ignorant and cruel. Religious communities might be more attractive if their members could toss out the rotten apples.

Yet she argues that a religious community is not simply a sanctimonious country club—a collection of like-minded people handpicked by an inner circle. It is more like a family whose members are, as Daniel says, "stuck with one another." The curious fact about family is that its members are forced to interact in too close a proximity to mask their idiosyncrasies and shortcomings. "When you are stuck with one another," Daniel says, "the last thing you would do is invent a God based on humanity. . . . In community, humanity is just way too close to look good."

It seems odd that in the twenty-first century people would voluntarily commit to a group they cannot choose for the sake of some other good. It seems odd that people like Daniel would prescribe such a commitment as an antidote to an individual's personally crafted spirituality. But the fact of the matter is that people have been choosing to belong to religious communities for most of human existence.

Why do people do this? Why do they insist on committing to communities of otherwise disparate persons united primarily by a particular system of faith and worship? Daniel's answer, which is likely the answer for most religious people, is that there are aspects of their particular systems of faith and worship that completely transform them as individuals and as communities. And for many, that transformation links directly to questions of meaning and purpose in life and death—and after death.

An Ancient Debate

In the ancient world, no one escaped death. Most cultures were crystal clear that the dead did not rise again. All kinds of other things could happen to the dead, of course. Plato and his followers were convinced that the soul departed the body at death—so-called Platonic dualism. Others thought that souls of the deceased occasionally appeared to human mortals. Still others believed that the souls of the dead dwelt among the tombs.

Despite these views, no so-called pagan in late antiquity believed that a soul would eventually take on a restored body. That is, no polytheist believed in the resurrection of the dead. But many Jews did. And later Christians—whose beliefs were rooted in Judaism—also did.

Jon Levenson, Harvard professor of Jewish studies, has repeatedly drawn attention to what he calls "a central belief in rabbinic Judaism" that has received scant notice in the modern day. That belief is the resurrection, the idea that God will revive the dead at the end of history and will "restore them to full bodily existence."

Some Jewish groups in late antiquity, such as the Sadducees, rejected the idea of the resurrection. Indeed, it is not central to Hebrew scripture. But most first-century Jews believed that the end of time would be marked by a general resurrection of the dead. Some thought that all would be resurrected; others believed that only God's chosen people would be resurrected. No Jewish person at the time understood resurrection to be possible prior to that ultimate general resurrection of the dead.

The suggestion that the dead would eventually come alive again in restored bodies was not some peripheral, secondary belief. According to Levenson, it was "a weight-bearing beam in the edifice of rabbinic Judaism." It strengthened the rabbinic notion of redemption and Jewish personhood. As Levenson puts it, "Without the restoration of the people Israel, a flesh-and-blood people, God's promises to them remained unfulfilled, and the world remained unredeemed." There was no sidelining this doctrine. The future of the Jewish people depended on it.

The first "Christ followers," or Christians, were Jewish because Jesus was Jewish, and they embraced the Jewish conception of the resurrection. But three days after Jesus was crucified—as depicted so graphically by Grünewald's altarpiece—his followers began to proclaim the radical idea that Jesus had risen from the dead. This uprooted deep cultural assumptions; resurrection was not supposed to happen prior to that final general resurrection.

In fact, after the death and reported resurrection of Jesus, the idea of resurrection itself shifted markedly. It went from being a vague notion that people would one day rise again as embodied persons to a concrete assertion that a new body with new properties would be created from old material. Resurrection went from functioning as a metaphor for the restoration of Israel to a metaphor for baptism. More than this, however, the radical claim that Jesus rose from the dead inspired hope in his followers. Death would not have the final word.

When I met Edith Blatchley that day in the hospital, she was dying and she knew it. In the moments I spoke with her, she was acutely aware of her own finitude and of her reluctance to face it squarely. What the nurses perceived to be a feistiness and lack of cooperation was, in reality, a cry for help, a last-ditch effort to reckon with the religious questions that plagued her.

Edith's experience is not unique to those who are actively dying. On some level, her story characterizes our culture's efforts to avoid death altogether. As a medical doctor, I have watched patients push off questions of death time and time again. It is difficult for the Ediths of the world to die well when they go to the grave haunted by questions they consistently chose to ignore. In failing to die well, we fail to live well. By avoiding questions of the meaning of death, we avoid questions of the meaning of life. By avoiding finitude, we ignore infinitude.

When we think of Ms. Blatchley, we may feel sorry for her, alone in the hospital ward, clutching her sheet over her emaciated body, failing to rest in peace.

Vandalized *Shalom*

Why are we, like Ms. Blatchley, evading questions that irk us? Levenson provides one answer with regard to the ancient Jewish commitment to the resurrection. He says that many Jews—although certainly not all—have adopted a strategic posture, downplaying the resurrection in order to keep from being assimilated into a dominant Christian culture. Moreover, "by excluding the resurrection of the dead from Judaism," Levenson writes, "modern Jews can appear to the world and, more important, to themselves as simultaneously adhering to a way of thinking that is as old and particular as the Hebrew Bible and as new and universal as modern science." Modern beliefs for modern Jews.

Could this be true for most of us? Do we conceive of "all that religion nonsense" as part of a fundamentally outmoded way of thinking and living? Do we feel compelled by the demands of modernity to shirk the beliefs of traditional religious communities?

Lillian Daniel certainly thinks that this is the case. She blames the West's secular consumer culture for elevating a do-it-yourself spirituality and denigrating the importance of religious community. For Daniel, not only does modern life squelch our "Why?" questions; it thwarts the assembly of the very communities that help us make sense of such questions. And who knows? When it comes to death and an afterlife, the stakes might be high.

Levenson and coauthor Kevin Madigan argue that in

the West today there remains little to console the twenty-first-century public in the face of death. They write: "When the emphasis lies on the individual and his or her power of self-determination, as it generally does in modern Western thought, then the loss of the individual to death will inevitably seem catastrophic and irreversible." But the authors do not end there. They add a parenthetical statement: "The loss of the individual to death will inevitably seem catastrophic and irreversible (unless, of course, it can be reversed through resurrection)." For Levenson and Madigan, as for so many ancient Jews and Christians, the redemption of the catastrophic—that is, the hope in death—depends entirely on death's reversal.

Today biomedicine has taken up the mantle of providing hope in death. In this modern age, when the dead body is a broken machine and the spiritually curious can create their own belief systems, health-care professionals have stepped into the gap. No longer considered healers, we are called "providers"— the purveyors of death-delaying goods to our consumer patients. We deliver hope through pills and infusions, working tirelessly to reverse the effects of aging, disease, and death. And we often succeed. But even when we resuscitate the same Mr. Turner three times in one night, our best work ultimately fails. The universe seems stacked against us.

People often ask me why I am so interested in writing on death. Yes, I have lost close friends and family members to devastating disease. And yes, I have cared for countless patients battling mortality in myriad ways. These experiences have certainly shaped me. But more than this, I am intrigued by the questions patients ask for which modern medicine has no solution—questions many doctors try to avoid. I don't pretend to have easy answers, but I am willing to "go there" with my patients. And somehow, these conversations—imbued with mystery and fear—transform our relationships. I cease to be a "provider"—what good or service can I possibly provide? Instead, I again become a physician, a healer who aspires to see her patients flourish.

Broken bodies, broken communities, a broken world—a friend of mine calls this "vandalized *shalom*." *Shalom*, the Hebrew word for "peace," refers to peace in its most robust sense: wholeness, harmony, flourishing. Vandalized peace, my friend says, means not just laboring to build the boat but striving to bail the boat, which has sprung leaks everywhere. Removing a cancerous tumor should bring *shalom*. But vandalized *shalom* means not just having the tumor removed, but striving to stay afloat amidst the complications of surgery, the side effects of chemotherapy, and the frustrations of a prolonged hospital stay.

It is not my aim here to offer a tidy solution to vandalized *shalom*, but simply to raise the possibility that dying wisely might require us to wrestle with some tough questions that we, like Ms. Blatchley, have ignored our whole lives. Dying well means grappling with our existential questions and not avoiding them. The *ars moriendi* attends to the metaphysical as well as the physical.

Existential answers take a variety of forms. For some, as we have seen, the answer might lie in online courses on transcending transpersonal realms. Others might find that SBNR is insufficient and return to the ancient beliefs of their religious forebears. Still others, like the poet Christian Wiman in Chapter Five, struggle with it all and yet somehow find that they believe.

Wiman characterizes himself in his earlier years as an "ambivalent atheist" who struggled with "an inchoate loneliness and endless anxieties." But at some point he "found faith," which he says is fundamentally different from religion. Although now a church regular, Wiman remains ambivalent about religion, its institutions, and "the whole goddamned shebang." But he cannot stop himself from believing. He writes:

One doesn't follow God in hope of happiness but because one senses . . . a truth that renders ordinary contentment irrelevant. There are some hungers that only an endless commitment to emptiness can feed, and the only true antidote to the plague of modern despair is an absolute, and perhaps even annihilating, awe. "I asked for wonders instead of happiness, Lord," writes the Jewish theologian Abraham Joshua Heschel. "And you gave them to me."

I asked for wonders instead of happiness, and you gave them to me.

CHAPTER EIGHT

RITUAL

Ricky Mitchell was a seventy-five-year-old lifelong smoker who, after numerous hospitalizations for exacerbation of his emphysema, decided that he had had enough. During his previous six or seven hospital stays, his lungs had been so weak that his doctors had inserted a breathing tube into his airway and connected him to the mechanical ventilator in the intensive-care unit. Each time it took longer and longer to wean him off the ventilator.

During his most recent hospital stay, he reached the maximum allowable time for a breathing tube. In order to prevent damage to the back of the throat, called the larynx, Mr. Mitchell's medical team advised that he receive a tracheostomy, a hole in the neck through which a ventilator would connect to his airway. Although it was possible that his lungs might eventually improve enough to allow the tracheostomy to be removed, his doctors remained doubtful.

Mr. Mitchell would have none of it. He was intubated, so he could not speak. But on a piece of paper he scrawled the following words: "Would rather die than live on machine. Made my peace." And with this declaration, the ritual of removing the endotracheal tube began.

Pulling the Plug

Death creates chaos on every level—emotional, existential, practical. There are questions of decorum. Is it acceptable to weep with joy if death offers an end to suffering? And how much happiness is permissible during those first postmortem days? There also linger countless unanswered existential questions. Why did she have to suffer? Why the untimely death? Where is God? What's more, the finality of death itself triggers a host of pragmatic issues about which decisions must be made. Autopsy? Funeral home? Casket? Cremation? Burial plot? Service? Guests? Flowers? Estate? Recovering the deceased's frequent flyer miles?

Out of this vandalized *shalom* emerges *ritual*—the orderly, tradition-based, formal performances that accompany our most profound events—what the columnist David Brooks calls "social architecture that marks and defines life's phases." Although ancient rituals have lost the cultural cachet they once possessed, ritual remains central to the recovery of an art of dying.

Generally speaking, rituals engage community to unite matters of body and spirit. Rituals mark rites of passage—coming of age, graduation, marriage. They provide time-tested scripts when unprecedented change upends our carefully constructed lives. At the very least, death-related rituals offer us a road map for what to do when a living person becomes a corpse. Ritual describes how we are to accompany the dead body to its final rest.

The modern secular hospital has created its own rituals surrounding death. Like Mr. Mitchell, many of my patients tell me that if they are "too far gone" (a rather loosely defined limit), they want me "to pull the plug"—that ritual of removing life support, often a mechanical ventilator.

The ceremonial act of "pulling the plug" adheres to a prescribed order and formality. In Mr. Mitchell's case, the head of the medical team met with him and his wife to establish that he was of sound mind and to confirm his request. A convincing Mr. Mitchell clearly restated his wish to discontinue life support, acknowledging that this might in fact lead to his death.

The doctor informed the Mitchell family that sometimes doctors get it wrong; on rare occasions patients survive for years after removal of the breathing tube. No one was trying to kill him by disconnecting life support, and no one was guaranteeing his death. However, it was highly likely that he would have difficulty breathing, and the medical team promised to do everything in its power to prevent his gasping for breath. When all questions had been answered satisfactorily, Mr. Mitchell's family notified their broader community.

The next step in the ritual is providing opportunity for loved ones to say farewell. With a somber air, family and friends began to file slowly into the intensive-care unit, bringing flowers, favorite photographs, music, and other mementos they wished to share with their beloved Mr. Mitchell before his breathing tube was removed. They sat at his bedside, offered their apologies for various bygones, and accepted his apologies for the same. They traded stories, took pictures, and sang songs. Someone recited a prayer. When they were ready, they signaled to the medical team.

The doctors then arrived at Mr. Mitchell's room and explained what would happen. They would give him just a little bit of morphine, so that his breathing would not be labored. He would remain alert and fully conscious. They reiterated to those gathered at the bedside that all prior attempts to remove the tube had failed, and they doubted he would breathe well without it. Still there remained a chance that Mr. Mitchell might breathe on his own without the tube. They assured the family that the morphine would not end his life but would provide some relief for potentially labored breathing. Under no circumstances would the doctors hasten his death once the tube was out.

When everyone was ready, the nurses suctioned the tube to remove excess phlegm from Mr. Mitchell's airway. Then they ceremoniously unfastened the exterior strap holding the tube in place and deflated a small balloon that helped to maintain the tube's position inside the trachea. As the ventilator forced a breath into his lungs, the doctors pulled the tube out. They then gave him an oxygen mask to ease any sensation of air hunger.

The next moments are the most intense for the ritual's observers, because there is no predicting what will happen. Will he resume spontaneous breathing or not? For a patient like Mr. Mitchell, whose lungs are in such bad shape, death almost always ensues.

As he labored to breathe, the nurses administered small doses of morphine to take the edge off. His lungs lacked the strength to continue on their own. Over minutes, his heart rate and breathing gradually slowed. And then his breathing stopped. Mr. Mitchell was dead.

Then a new ritual ensued: the declaration of death. As Amit and I did that night for Mr. Turner after his third death, a doctor on the medical team shone a penlight into Mr. Mitchell's eyes confirming that the pupils would not constrict. She placed her stethoscope on his chest to confirm that the heartbeats and breaths had stopped. These gestures complete, she offered her condolences to Mr. Mitchell's wife and family and excused herself to complete the death certificate, concluding the ritual.

The family sat for more than an hour and grieved with the body. After they left the intensive-care unit, the nurses covered Mr. Mitchell's body with a sheet, and it was delivered headfirst to the morgue, where it would remain until released for funerary rituals, typically under the guidance of a funeral director.

When Mr. Mitchell died, his wife called the funeral director, who in turn called the embalmer. In most states, the funeral director arranges for the deceased's final disposition, and a licensed embalmer prepares the body. In some states the funeral director also embalms. Mr. Mitchell's body was collected from the hospital morgue and embalmed for the viewing, funeral, and burial, which took place the following week.

For those not wishing to be embalmed, the funeral director may arrange for cremation. Cremation rates vary widely around the world. In the United States today, about half of bodies are cremated, although that number is climbing due to the high cost of burial. In the United Kingdom, as a comparison, roughly three-quarters of bodies are cremated. In Japan, nearly 100 percent of the deceased are cremated, while other countries such as Serbia and Ghana cremate fewer than 10 percent. Religious and cultural practices play a deciding role—Muslim- and Catholic-majority countries are more inclined to bury bodies whole, whereas countries with large Hindu or Buddhist populations tend toward cremation.

Preparing a Body

Jenn Park-Mustacchio is a licensed funeral director and embalmer in New Jersey. At the time of her interview with the *Guardian*, she worked primarily in embalming. The deceased's relative would call the funeral home, and the funeral director would notify Park-Mustacchio. Then her day would start.

Embalming has been practiced for thousands of years; the ancient Egyptians were perhaps its most famous practitioners. Although shallow graves and desert heat provided the perfect conditions for natural mummification, the Egyptians believed that embalming was a ritual necessary for successful tenure in the afterlife. They perfected the process. Although it has changed a little over the millennia, the final effect has not.

Today's embalmers follow their own sets of rituals. Park-Mustacchio describes a multistep process for preparing a body that has died a "typical" death. She begins by suiting up in protective gear, donning the gown, apron, gloves, and shoe covers of a modern-day embalmer. Next she "sets the features," closing eyes and mouth and arranging limbs. She then infuses the embalming fluid, uniquely prepared for each corpse based on weight and height. As the fluid flows through the body, the deceased's blood drains out of a large vein.

Next Park-Mustacchio massages the body with a soapy sponge, which helps with drainage of the blood and distribution of the embalming fluid. In time the fluid improves the corpse's coloring, and she cuts off the fluid infusion and instills a stronger fluid in the body's hollow cavities. Finally, she washes and dresses the corpse, applying cream to the face to prevent the skin from drying out.

Park-Mustacchio finds fulfillment in her work. It is especially satisfying, she says, when a difficult case turns out better than expected and a family commends her work or decides to have an open instead of a closed casket. "The best compliment I got was from a woman whose daughter died of bone cancer. She took my hand and said, 'Thank you. She's so beautiful, she looks like she could get up and dance.'"

Most of us, at least the North Americans among us, are probably grateful for embalmers like Park-Mustacchio, who not only take pride in their work but literally *undertake* the tasks that most of us would be reluctant to perform. But does it not strike us as odd that the care of the body of a deceased loved one would be assigned to the next available on-call embalmer?

And why embalm a body anyway? Is it a necessary ritual? The journalist Jessica Mitford, perhaps best known for her exposé of the funeral industry, *The American Way of Death*, notes that beyond the United States and Canada almost no one embalms. No law or religion requires embalming, she notes, "nor is it dictated by considerations of health, sanitation, or even of personal daintiness." Most people fail to realize that with attention to certain state laws, it is possible to have an open casket at a funeral without embalming the deceased.

Embalming became big business in the United States in the 1860s during the Civil War. Unprecedented numbers of soldiers died. When possible, the bodies of the deceased were sent back to their families by train, and it proved necessary to preserve the corpses for these long journeys. President Abraham Lincoln was an early champion of embalming. In 1862, his eleven-year-old son, Willie, died and was embalmed by the same team that would embalm the assassinated president three years later.

Putting aside the question of whether to embalm (which I advise interested readers to explore further), I wish to return to the theme of caring for the bodies of the dead. The question is this: Whether or not we embalm, is it not curious that we willingly pass off responsibility for intimate rituals associated with attending to dead bodies? Shouldn't we be the ones to care for the bodies of our loved ones? Many of us, professional embalmers included, will be quick to point out that the work of embalming requires particular skill and emotional fortitude—it's definitely not for everyone. But in response it is worth noting that professionalizing the care of the dead is a relatively modern phenomenon.

Rituals develop from *within* communities for communities. They provide road maps through periods of great change or upheaval. This is why preceding generations have developed elaborate rituals for accompanying a body to its final rest. The Jewish ritual called *tahara* exemplifies this well, and I introduce it in order to highlight both what modern practices have lost and what modern rituals could once again become. Consider the contrast between *tahara* and the daily work of Park-Mustacchio.

Tahara

Although Jewish law forbids embalming, the body must still be prepared for burial. *Tahara* is the ritual of cleansing a dead body prior to burial. It underscores the concept of dignity that is central to Jewish rituals of birth, coming of age, and marriage. Just as a newborn baby is washed of the detritus of birth before its presentation, so too is the dead body prepared and "purified" for burial.

Tahara is performed by members of the *chevra kadisha*, or burial society (lit., "holy society"), a specially trained group of volunteers from within the Jewish community. Men attend to a male body and women to a female body. This gender-based division of labor hardly comes as a surprise; cultural practices with roots in the premodern era often divide this way. But what might surprise us is that those tasked with performing *tahara* actually speak to the body. There is no professional distancing—no anonymizing this work. They address the body by its Hebrew name and ask forgiveness in advance for any indignity they might inadvertently inflict on account of their work.

The members of the *chevra kadisha* begin by washing the body with warm water, not cold, as if it can feel. They carefully attend to every detail—fingernails, toenails, ear canals—as in the care of any living person. They maintain modesty by covering the body with a sheet, uncovering only the part they are washing.

Even more distinct from the way Park-Mustacchio prepares the dead is the holy love song that the society sings while it works. Borrowing the intimate poetry of the Hebrew Song of Songs, men sing to the male body and women to the female, "His head is the finest gold; his locks are wavy, black as a raven. His eyes are like doves beside springs of water." Then follows a second washing with cold water. Finally, they remove the sheet entirely and either immerse the body in a ritual bath, called a *mikveh*, or rinse it under a continuous stream of cool water. Then the body is dried, dressed in a shroud, and placed in the casket. The casket is not to be opened again. Honoring the dignity of the dead requires that no one look upon a body that cannot look back.

Catherine Madsen, of the Yiddish Book Center, notes that this ritual developed at a time in human history that had not yet been shaped by modern assumptions. There was, she says, "no Freud, no television, no concealment of death, no secularity anywhere." Our own prevailing squeamishness about death had not yet been cultivated. This meant that the lines from Song of Songs made possible a sort of freedom and sensitivity of expression and action that might not otherwise be possible in cleansing a dead body. Indeed, when I asked one of our local rabbis, Eliana Falk, how she might describe *tahara*, she answered with one word: "Love."

The practice of *tahara* today may vary slightly by local custom, and some Jewish funeral homes do not routinely offer it. But many are working to change this. Madsen's own synagogue identified a lack and set about to study the *tahara*. They formed a *chevra kadisha*. Reflecting on the experience of preparing a body, she notes that some members found the verses from Song of Songs "striking and powerful," while others "thought them obsolete and embarrassing." But the practice of reciting poetry helped the members of her *chevra kadisha* articulate complex and bewildering emotions associated with death. Madsen goes on:

If the lines had not been in the ritual, we would still have felt tenderness—one cannot handle the dead kindly without feeling tenderness—but we would have felt it inarticulately, perhaps only prompted to murmur on the way out that the occasion felt "very spiritual." Because the lines were there—because others had thought on that tenderness as profoundly as a profound tradition allows—we could be fully perceiving members of the tradition at the boundary line of perception. We could be fully alive on behalf of the dead.

Madsen believes that if proposed as a new ritual today, *tahara* would likely never be tolerated. "There would be nervous giggles about homoeroticism and necrophilia; the plan would be hotly discussed at one or two committee meetings, roundly declared inappropriate, and quietly dropped," she says.

But perhaps this is hyperbolic. There seems to be a growing interest among members of the Jewish community in modernizing ancient rituals. The acclaimed writer Anita Diamant, for example, established in Boston a "reinvented" *mikveh*, or ritual bath, where individuals can immerse themselves to mark a fresh start after trauma, graduation, divorce, or chemotherapy. On the opposite coast, Rabbi Avivah Erlick founded Sacred Waters, which performs a personalized *tahara* in the homes or care facilities of nontraditional Jews and even of non-Jews who might adopt Jewish death rituals.

For all of us—Jewish or not, religious or secular—such rituals should prompt questions about how we might honor the bodies of the deceased. Should we prepare bodies ourselves within our communities, without receiving thanks or payment? Is something lost by handing the task off to a professional? Can ancient texts imbue meaning in a dying process that has otherwise become medicalized and secularized? What does it mean for us to be fully alive on behalf of the dead?

Funeral as Theater

Since the beginning, the dead have demanded respect. Although it is a paradox to imagine the dead demanding anything, they nevertheless captivate us despite their silence. When Princess Diana died in 1997, she held the undivided attention of some 1 million mourners lining the processional route, with another 2.5 billion television viewers following from a distance.

The dead inspire awe and quiet reverence. But death also induces in its survivors a state of helplessness. Shocked by the blow of human loss, many become unable to make decisions clearly. This death-induced state of vulnerability is precisely why community leaders over the years have given so much care not only to preparing the dead body but also to the rituals associated with laying that body to rest. This is why the *ars moriendi* developed in the first place.

Before I started writing about practices at the end of life, I had not given much thought to why certain customs had developed. My B-17 bomber pilot grandfather had raised me to think that death requires a coffin, hearse, funeral service, and cemetery plot. From my earliest memories, he was always talking—joking even—about his death. War can do that to a person, especially to a grandfather famous for his sense of humor. Over the years, however, I began to learn that, with regard to funerals, much more is required than a coffin and hearse.

The most fantastic element of a funeral is that it should be theater—a community performance. For many people, the idea of funeral as theater sounds insincere and disrespectful—even "debased," to use the description of theater by the great acting instructor Stella Adler. Theater, we might assume, is mere entertainment. It's about triggering the right emotions in the audience—isn't it?

The word *theater* comes from the Greek meaning "a place for viewing," or as Adler puts it, "the seeing place." The theater, she says, is where people see or discover truths about life and society. Sometimes these truths are explored through comedy, but a funeral is more akin to a great drama with a solemn message—a story with a moral to it. In his book on funerals Thomas Long says that they are neither entertainment nor "mere inspiration, but a deep probing into the things that make us or break us as human beings." Funerals should provide for us an opportunity to "see" our own finitude.

Earlier we discussed dying-as-drama through the story of the seventeenth-century French courtier Madame de Montespan. By supporting Madame in her dying, her servants also rehearsed for their own deaths. And this is precisely what the drama of a funeral is meant to do. Long says that the funeral is not only performed *for* the community; it is performed *by* the community. Everybody present has a role to play. "The purpose of a funeral is not to uplift the audience," he says, "but to transform the cast."

How should funerals transform us, the cast members? Long identifies two questions by which we might assess a "good" funeral. The first asks how well the funeral helps people to see what he calls "a truth worth seeing." The second concerns the degree to which the funeral invites its actors to play their parts and thereby be transformed, "to go beyond preoccupations with self, and to move toward that larger, redemptive truth that lies outside of them."

These are questions of seeing and of responding to what is seen. These are the questions of theater. Indeed, Long takes his cues here from Adler herself, who tells her aspiring actors, "You have to get beyond your own precious inner experiences now. I want you to be able to see and share what you see with an audience, not just get wrapped up in yourself." It is vital, she says, that actors look beyond themselves. "The ideas of the great playwrights are almost always larger than the experiences of even the best actors," Adler concludes.

Just what are we to see in a funeral? What larger stories are represented?

The Queen and the Maverick

It just so happened that as I was writing this chapter Americans lost two heroes. Aretha Franklin, the "Queen of Soul," died of pancreatic cancer on August 16, 2018, and the "maverick" senator John McCain died of brain cancer on August 25, 2018. Although their communities and the nation mourned their deaths and celebrated their lives over many days, their funerals took place within twenty-four hours of one another. Both hailed from Christian backgrounds, so I was particularly intrigued to see how their funerals represented some of Christianity's larger stories.

Thomas Long says that all elements of the central Christian funeral rite are imbued with meaning—they point to a much larger story. In his book he combs through a wide range of Christian funeral traditions—Catholic, Protestant, and Eastern Orthodox—to give us what he posits are the features that unite them.

Take, for example, the presence of the body at a funeral. Most Christian funerals over time have taken place in churches, the common weekly meeting place for the faithful. But what sets the funeral apart from other meetings is the fact that among those gathered is the one who just died. As Long puts it, "This saint, though deceased, is still joined to the congregation and is coming in the body to this place one last time for worship." In contrast to the notion that funerals are for the living—that they exist to meet the needs of mourners—Long argues that funerals are for both the living and the dead.

It's something like a wedding, he says. The community gathers—traditionally in a church—to mark a major life transition corporately. But no one would gather for a wedding without the bride and groom. Likewise, no one gathers at a funeral without the presence of the deceased.

This point is driven home by the dramatic arrival of the body of the dead. Once the community has gathered in the church, the pallbearers either carry or escort (on a cart) the inhabited coffin from the entrance of the church down its central aisle.

Some traditions enhance the procession symbolically. For example, clergy may lead with a cross or a candle meant to symbolize the light of Christ in the world. Others require that the priest or minister walk in front of the coffin while speaking of the resurrection and Christian hope. As the body passes by, the congregation might sing a hymn as a reminder of their shared story—that death is ultimately powerless, that resurrection of the body awaits.

The procession of the dead is meant to represent the last time that the deceased takes his or her place in the assembly for worship. Because of this, some traditions hold that laypeople are carried feetfirst, facing the front, as they would have entered the church any week when living. By contrast, deceased clergy are carried headfirst so as to face the congregation as they would have when presiding over a service.

At most of the church funerals I have attended, the coffin is placed in the front center of the church, parallel to the pews. This means that the pallbearers must turn a sharp right or left when they arrive at the front of the church. But this isn't the traditional place to put the coffin. Although a funeral is in some sense theater, older convention dictates that the coffin is not to be displayed in the front of the church. Rather, the deceased is meant symbolically to participate, for the last time, in communal worship. And to do so requires that the dead person be "seated" or positioned in the aisle between the front pews, in the midst of the congregation.

In reality, people do all kinds of things. Aretha Franklin's coffin arrived well in advance of her funeral at Detroit's Greater Grace Temple, accompanied by her pallbearers. She was placed prominently in the front center of the church auditorium, parallel to the front pews, and just in front of the central pulpit. The queen was set apart, open casket on display. But importantly, she was still on the same level as her friends and family who had gathered in a final act of worship.

Although Franklin did not make the conventional grand entrance down the central aisle in the midst of a seated congregation, her community processed past her to pay its final respects. In fact, the first ninety minutes of her funeral were given over to the solemn sight of hundreds of mourners processing silently down the central aisle, pausing to gaze at Franklin's lifeless form. Some whispered words. Some crossed their chests. It was theater in the best sense of the word.

At John McCain's official funeral, held at the Washington National Cathedral, an honor guard accompanied the coffin down the center aisle to the front. The coffin was placed on a bier in the middle of the center aisle—not in the midst of the congregation, but in front of it, below the altar. As with the queen, the maverick was set apart.

None Shall Sleep

The funerals of both Franklin and McCain broke in small ways with tradition, yet neither lost the opportunity to remind those in attendance of their larger story. In that "seeing place" of the funerary theater, the messages were difficult to ignore.

As the congregation paraded past Franklin's body, the choir belted out "Marvelous" by famed Gospel singer Walter Hawkins, recounting their shared narrative of liberation through Jesus:

> You gave that I might live
> You gave that I might be set free
> Exchanged your life for mine
> What a Marvelous thing you've done

The song recounts the teaching that the faithful are set free from the bondage of sin by the sacrifice of Christ—the "you" in the song. It serves to remind the living that even though all die a physical death—the bodies of the queen and the maverick are buried in the ground—Christ's resurrection should inspire hope in death's impermanence.

The Dallas megachurch pastor T. D. Jakes drove this message home when he stepped up to the pulpit for one of the readings. He began with a story, recounting the time in 1998 when he and his wife first attended the Grammy awards. Luciano Pavarotti was scheduled to perform that night but fell ill. "And guess who took his place?" Jakes asked. "Aretha Franklin—with class and dignity."

Franklin sang that night "with finesse and power and clarity." She enchanted the audience with the popular aria from Giacomo Puccini's opera *Turandot*, "Nessun Dorma," which means "none shall sleep." Jakes continued: "And even though it appears that she is laying in a box, the song is true. None shall sleep. She is not here, she has risen." This was the point of Jakes's story, the truth that the bereaved were to see in that seeing place.

The choir, the preachers, and the readings rehearsed this story again and again during Franklin's nine-hour funeral, just as they did at McCain's. As McCain's coffin was carried down the church's center aisle, the priest solemnly recited "The Burial of the Dead: Rite Two" from the *Book of Common Prayer*:

> I am Resurrection and I am Life, says the Lord.
> Whoever has faith in me shall have life,
> even though he die.
> And everyone who has life,
> and has committed himself to me in faith,
> shall not die for ever.

This is the substance of the larger drama of the Christian funeral. "Though he die, he shall not die for ever." Death but not death. Death and then life. This is the story that the deceased's community—the actors of the drama—are invited to inhabit.

Ritual does not exist for its own sake, but to establish order during rites of passage and major life disruptions by pointing toward a truth worth pursuing and by animating community members to respond to that truth.

Between Grief and Consolation

Rabbi Eliana Falk says that of all the things Judaism does well, it does death the best. And from what I have seen, she's right.

The rabbis of the Talmud established a series of phases of mourning within Judaism. The idea is that grief diminishes with the passing of time, and thus the ritual obligations and expectations for the bereaved vary with distance from death. Right after someone dies, it's all hands on deck. The community fully supports the grieving for a week or so and then gradually backs off.

Perhaps the simplest way to think about grief in the Jewish tradition is to divide its phases according to a timeline:

- The time from death to burial, usually one day, is called *aninut*.
- The first seven days after burial are called *shivah*.
- The first thirty days after burial are called *sheloshim*.
- The anniversary of the death is called by its Yiddish name, *yahrzeit*.

These stages follow the natural progression from initial shock, to a period of receiving condolences and community support, to the gradual reentry into normal life. *Yahrzeit* concludes the twelve months of mourning, and the bereaved are to weep no more.

Doctors today believe that it generally takes people a full year to get back to "life as usual" after they experience the loss of a loved one. As these ancient mourning rituals indicate, the Jewish tradition figured out therapeutic grieving long before present-day psychologists did.

For the purpose of our consideration of ritual, it is worth focusing specifically on what *shivah* can teach us. The word *shivah* literally means "seven"—the first seven days of mourning from the time of burial. Some people refer to it as "sitting *shivah*," because of the mourners' custom of sitting on low stools or on the floor in the home. The idea comes from the biblical book of Job; after Job lost his family and almost everything he owned, his friends sat with him on the ground for seven days and seven nights, mourning in solidarity.

The bereaved are to do no work during the week of *shivah*. No one cooks or leaves the house—visitors bring all necessary food provisions. *Shivah* is a time for weeping and not for concern with personal appearances. In many houses the mirrors are covered to underscore the point that *shivah* is for reflecting on the dead and not on the self. Some mourners refrain from shaving, wearing makeup, and showering. The wound of death is raw and deep—the bereaved are expected to do nothing other than to sit and mourn. According to the classic code of Jewish law, visitors to a home observing *shivah* are not to speak unless the mourner speaks; this is no occasion for small talk. And visitors are to leave when directed by the mourner.

Rabbi Falk told me that it wasn't until her parents died that she realized just how profound an experience sitting *shivah* can be: "Throughout each afternoon and evening, callers walked quietly into the house, and sat with us. They accompanied us, sometimes wordlessly, as it is the custom not to offer words of comfort when a loss is so new and deeply felt."

At other times, visitors would listen as Falk and her family reminisced about the one who had died. "This was an opportunity," she said, "for us to begin the new practice of keeping the memories of their joys and challenges alive." Jewish and non-Jewish friends, family members, neighbors, and even people she didn't know came to offer the gift of physical presence, joining in prayer services together each evening.

Shivah prepared and equipped Falk to move forward: "The awesome power of the unity of all present—both in life and in spirit, created a space rich in life-affirming love, hope and the promise of healing and resilience. At the end of the seven days of *shivah*, we were prepared to walk out into a new phase of life knowing that our faith, tradition, family, and friends would support us."

I found myself pondering these mourning phases after a close friend lost her mother rather unexpectedly. When my friend texted the news, I knew that she had already entered the intense period of *aninut*—marked by consuming grief combined with a host of burial obligations. Although she did not specifically follow Talmudic mourning practices, she opened the family home during the first week after her mother's death to a constant stream of relatives and friends who aimed to accompany the family. The acuity of loss faded into a raw wound in subsequent weeks, and family members resumed life as usual. It was not until about day thirty, almost precisely the end of *sheloshim*, that my friend contacted me to meet again as was our routine. I was struck that her grieving seemed to align almost precisely with Jewish phases of grief.

The renowned British rabbi Jonathan Sacks says that Jewish law aims at the midpoint between too much and too little grief. He writes:

> We are commanded not to engage in excessive rituals of grief. To lose a close member of one's family is a shattering experience. It is as if something of ourselves had died too. Not to grieve is wrong, inhuman: Judaism does not command Stoic indifference in the face of death. But to give way to wild expressions of sorrow . . . is also wrong.

The phases of mourning in Judaism serve as a guide in the midst of chaos, gently leading mourners through the shocking numbness of initial loss. From within the embrace of community, the bereaved are permitted to mourn. And through the phases of mourning they are slowly accompanied back into daily life.

Today's modern hospital rituals, such as pulling the plug on Ricky Mitchell, lack the depth and communal emphasis that belong to more ancient traditions. Removing life support and embalming corpses offer the veneer of ritual, but they are technical, procedural, perfunctory. They are efficient, but efficiency does not allow the bereaved to see the truths worth seeing. Efficiency forces bodies onto conveyor belts, and conveyor belts move too quickly.

The rituals highlighted in this chapter are not exhaustive. There exist many other death-related customs and practices. But these described should prompt us to ask how best to care for and accompany the bodies of our departed loved ones. Rather than sidelining *tahara* or the funeral and mourning processes, we might instead explore and preserve them. In doing so, we give language and structure to the complex emotion that death arouses, and we become, as Madsen says, "fully perceiving members of the tradition at the boundary line of perception . . . fully alive on behalf of the dead."

As we seek to reinvigorate the *ars moriendi* today, it is worth asking ourselves how we might also reinvigorate ritual.

CHAPTER NINE

LIFE

Try as I might, I have never been able to forget an older man who waited patiently to speak with me one night after a lecture I gave in the Midwest. I don't remember now if he told me his age, but in my mind he was somewhere between seventy-eight and eighty-two. A retired medical doctor, he knew death better than most. Despite this, he had never experienced it firsthand—that is, he himself had never died—until very recently.

He beckoned me away from the crowd gathered at the podium and got right to the point. A few years earlier, he had needed open-heart surgery, and he had died on the operating table.

"What did you see?" I asked, sensing that this was what he

wished to discuss. Over the years I have heard many stories of near-death experiences—an inviting white light or familiar faces of relatives long deceased. One woman told me that when she suffered a heart attack and died, she left her body. She watched the doctors resuscitate her from some perch near the ceiling.

The old doctor was hesitating, so I asked him again. "What did you see?" A mishmash of curiosity, impatience, and post-lecture enthusiasm propelled my questioning.

"That's just the problem. I didn't see anything," he replied. "Nothing. Absolutely nothing." He paused. "And it frightened me."

His hushed tone, posture, and facial expressions said it all. He was petrified. And as he stood before me, twice my age, he wanted to know what he should do about it.

In all honesty, I had never met someone who had died, been resuscitated, and seen nothing. The most fervent atheist had seen *something*, even if some scientists explain it as the result of changes to the brain associated with normal dying. But nothing? Really *nothing*? I didn't have a ready answer.

Now it was my turn to pause. I did so, liberally. Then, wanting to ease his fear, I said, "Well, maybe you saw nothing, because you weren't ready to die. And now you have time to prepare."

Seeming to accept my words, he retreated.

Putting It All Together

If the *ars moriendi* teaches us anything, it's that the work of living well is what enables dying well. The tasks of living well include living each day in the context of community with a view to finitude. In this sense, the elderly doctor had not lived well. He had not lived with a view to his finitude. He had neither anticipated nor prepared for his death. He had not engaged questions of meaning and purpose within the context of a community that had wrestled with such questions. As a result, he feared that he would not die well.

But what I told him that night is true for each person holding this book now—you have time to prepare for death. And you had best start today.

What might it look like to live well in order to die well? In the preceding chapters I have attempted to lay this out, and a brief recap is called for as we move into this final chapter.

I began the book with a description of the three deaths and resuscitations of my patient Mr. Turner. Mr. Turner was a religious man with strong community ties, so we might be tempted to think that he had made his proverbial peace. But he and his family were not prepared for death from a practical standpoint, and he died a grisly, highly medicalized death. As I suggested in Chapter One, the *ars moriendi*, or "art of dying" booklets, were developed in response to the widespread sentiment that people were unprepared for death. And they have something to teach us.

Chapter Two explored further the art of dying through a meditation on human finitude. We have to acknowledge our humanness, our mortality, our *finitude*, if we want to die well. It's requisite, but it's not the only criterion, which is why Chapter Three made the case for living and dying within the embrace of vibrant communities, and Chapter Four challenged the hospital as preferred destination for death. Why not aim to die at home, if this is within the realm of possibility?

Chapters Five to Eight attempted to address head-on the questions that so many medical doctors avoid—fear of death, decay of bodies, spirit and afterlife, and the role of ritual. If these subjects are featured in an art of dying, they should be listed as first orders of business in any art of living. It turns out that you can't keep this stuff for the end.

I am struck that most of us approach the end of our lives having tackled some but not all of these issues, and in this final chapter I'd like to offer a concise and practical guide—a handbook, if you will—on how to live well in order to die well.

All of what follows builds on three assumptions. First, the *ars moriendi* provides a useful model for anticipating and preparing for death. Second, we cannot die well if we do not acknowledge our own finitude. Third, we cannot die well in isolation; it is vital to engage our broader communities. Any readers perplexed by these assumptions I refer back to the first three chapters of the book.

Thinking Twice About Hospitalization

As I make the rounds of my hospitalized patients, they often comment that they slept poorly—their slumber was disrupted by late night blood-pressure checks, early morning blood draws, or other noisy patients. Sometimes I joke gently in return that the hospital is no place for the sick. It's true, and my patients respond with a knowing chuckle.

If the hospital is no place for the sick—or for the dying, as we have discussed—then for whom does the hospital exist? My answer is that the hospital exists for the acutely ill. No one quibbles about the vital role played by emergency rooms. No one argues that complex surgeries should be performed else- where. And it goes without saying that hospitals should house intensive-care units for care of the critically ill. But what about the mildly sick and the definitively dying?

These days, people typically die in one of three ways. A lifetime of good physical health eventually leads to a slow, constant waning late in life, often accompanied by memory problems and physical deconditioning. Others do well until some point in life when a dramatic illness provokes a relatively swift decline, as with incurable cancer or massive heart attack. The third group of people are those with organ failure, such as congestive heart failure or COPD, which includes emphy- sema and chronic bronchitis. Periodic exacerbations require hospitalization for tune-ups, which become more frequent as patients decline.

The first two groups spend most of their lives outside the hospital but turn to it increasingly as frailty or cancer takes over. The third group—those with organ failure—can spend decades in and out of the hospital, not quite realizing that the interval between hospitalizations shortens as the disease progresses. The result is that the hospital becomes the default destination for physical decline. And in the hospital, as we saw in Chapter One, conveyor-belt medicine automatically takes over.

The question, then, is: At what point should we stop going to the hospital? When is enough? I have pondered this for years now and routinely discuss it with my patients. For a long time I felt that people in their eighties should think twice before going to the hospital, and folks in their nineties should try to avoid it at all costs. But we all know eighty-eight-year-olds who still work full-time and play tennis regularly, and seventy-eight-year-olds who require around-the-clock nursing care. So age cutoffs aren't the answer. They are too simplistic.

Doctors increasingly turn to frailty assessments to help them determine who will benefit from a particular surgery or drug therapy and who might be harmed or even die from it. A frail person is one who does not bounce back easily from a minor stressor. A urinary tract infection that might cause painful urination and slight headache in a healthy older adult, for example, could trigger widespread infection and delirium in a frail elder. Many of us have an intuitive sense of frailty, but how do we say for sure who is frail? Determining frailty takes on greater importance if we are going to assert it as a criterion for forgoing hospitalization.

Medical researchers have come up with a variety of tools for measuring degree of frailty, but the assessment developed by the geriatrician Linda Fried and colleagues is perhaps the most widely used in the United States. It consists of five components; individuals are classified as "frail" if they are over sixty-five years of age and three or more of the following criteria apply:

- Unintentional weight loss of ten pounds or more in the last year
- Feelings of exhaustion
- Physical weakness, measured by checking handgrip strength with a dynamometer
- Slow walking speed, measured as requiring six or seven seconds to walk fifteen feet
- Low physical activity

I doubt that any reader has a dynamometer handy, but it's easy enough to notice when Grandpa can no longer hold his coffee mug or keep up with a leisurely stroll. It's also obvious when Grandpa's clothes have grown baggy and he spends all day napping. This is the stuff of frailty. And if you are sixty-five years of age and have three or more of these five characteristics, you too are likely frail.

Studies show that many factors besides old age put a person at risk for frailty. Intellectual disability, depression, smoking, and lower educational achievement all increase risk. In the United States, African Americans and Hispanics tend to have greater rates of frailty.

If you identify as frail, you are not the only one. When Fried applied her tool to a group of more than five thousand older men and women, she found that about 7 percent were frail. Another study found that among older cancer patients, 40 percent or more were frail. Many more can be classified as "prefrail," meaning that they meet one or two of the criteria for frailty.

Let's remember the point of all of these numbers. The more frail individuals are, the less likely they will recover well from even minor illnesses, not to mention major surgeries or prolonged hospitalizations. And for every day they spend in bed, they lose muscle mass, which is why hospitalizations as short as a few days often leave the elderly incredibly weak.

It is not uncommon for older patients to wish to remain longer in the hospital. They fear becoming sicker again at home and having to return. "Please, Doctor, just a couple more days here" is a common request from the elderly, even as they are starting to feel quite well again.

From the doctor's standpoint, however, we see how prolonged hospitalization leads not only to physical deconditioning and decreased strength, but also to increased risk of exposure to hospital-acquired infections. It may even lead to death itself. A group of Yale physicians found that among older hospitalized patients, those with poor physical function, poor nutrition, and dementia were much more likely to die in the hospital than those who easily attend to the activities of daily living such as bathing, toileting, dressing, walking, and eating. Hospitalization is not always the answer.

I have these sorts of conversations with my patients. Some of my very elderly patients—in their nineties and early hundreds—will probably never return to the hospital. They are so frail that no good can come of a hospitalization. To the extent possible, I even try to manage their medical care over the telephone, so as to avoid exposing them to other sick patients in my clinic.

I also have these conversations with my own family members. My grandparents moved to a senior complex when they were in their late eighties. As my grandfather declined, he moved to the nursing-home floor. At regular intervals, he would complain of abdominal pain or dizziness, and the staff would send him into the emergency room for an evaluation.

By the time he was in his early nineties, the entire family agreed that these frequent emergency-room visits for constipation and dizziness had to stop. What was Grandpa gaining apart from an opportunity to tell his jokes to a new audience? He had grown exceedingly frail, and there was no medical miracle in the world that would reverse this.

When thinking about family members, friends, or ourselves, it is wise to consider degree of frailty in order to avoid unnecessary procedures and hospital stays. But how are we to determine when a procedure or hospital stay is actually *unnecessary*?

Navigating Futile Treatments

Several years ago, a friend of mine died of metastatic cancer. At the time, we both had young children of similar ages, and our community included many young families. Despite walking with her through diagnosis, treatment, and relapse, all of us felt deeply the cruel sting of her premature death. It wounded us.

I was not her doctor, but as her friend it was my privilege to be able to help from time to time with some of the medical questions. I followed the ups and downs of her course as closely as I could. One Friday night her husband called to say that he thought she was dying.

"I think this is it," he said. "The cancer has invaded her liver. It is now three times normal size, and two-thirds of it is cancer. But her oncologist hasn't mentioned that she's dying." He told me that his wife was now completely yellow from jaundice. She herself declared that she was dying.

I figured that he was probably right. And since I had to be at the hospital early the next morning to check on my own patients, I promised to stop by their room as soon as I could.

Fortuitously, I made it to Beth's room just as her cancer doctors had gathered to discuss her clinical situation. I introduced myself, explained my relationship to the hospital as well as to the patient, and asked if I could listen in.

The conversation didn't last long. My friend's husband had nailed it—everyone on the team knew she was dying. Nothing more could be done.

I pulled the head oncologist aside before we entered the hospital room. "Her husband knows she's dying," I told the doctor. "He called me last night. Let's just see if we can get her home to be with her children." The oncologist agreed.

When I entered Beth's room, I was amazed at how little life remained. Thinned, yellowed, and weakened, she could hardly keep her head up and her eyes open. She seemed to pour every ounce of energy she could muster into her characteristically gracious welcome. She greeted us warmly before sinking back into her pillows.

The head oncologist sat down and reviewed the medical facts with my friends. She confirmed that they had read the signs well. The cancer was in fact consuming Beth's liver. That explained why she'd become so jaundiced.

"But—" The oncologist paused. I was waiting to hear how she would articulate to the young couple that Beth was dying. They were ready to hear it from the cancer doctor herself.

"But—" she said again. "There's one more medication we could try. A chemotherapy pill. She could take it at home. Theoretically it might have some benefit."

I was dumbfounded. All of the theoretical justification in the world could not obscure the obvious fact that my friend was dying. Her liver was dramatically and rapidly failing. If there were a chance in a million that she could live, she would have taken it—for her children's sake. But not now. It was too late. Beth knew it. We all knew it. So why didn't the oncologist tell her that she was dying? Why did she offer another drug?

The answer is common to many of the themes throughout this book. Doctors, like most other mortals, seek to avoid death, to thwart it. And sometimes it is easier to prescribe a pill than to tell a patient squarely that she is dying. The surgeon-writer Sherwin Nuland understands this. "Of all the professions, medicine is the one most likely to attract people with high personal anxieties about dying," he says. "We become doctors because our ability to cure gives us power over the death of which we are so afraid." By doing something—*anything*—doctors avoid difficult conversations.

So how are we to navigate this? Dying well requires preparation, and preparation requires an acknowledgment of human finitude. But if our own doctors pretend that we aren't dying, how are we to know when they are offering us treatments that are unlikely to be of benefit?

The first step in determining whether a treatment is futile is to take stock of frailty. In the case of my friend with cancer, there was no question that she met all five criteria for frailty mentioned above, despite her young age. A high degree of frailty should prompt some caution with regard to accepting new treatments.

But after taking stock, the next step is to press the doctor for meaningful answers to the tough questions. Doctors are accustomed to thinking through the risks and benefits—the bad and the good—of particular treatments. There is no reason not to insist on answers to questions such as, "How much is this going to help me?" and "What are the downsides of the treatment?"

And you can get specific. With regard to chemotherapy, you might ask, "Have you ever seen this drug help someone with my stage of cancer?" Or, "What is the likelihood that this treatment will make me so sick that I won't be able to enjoy the things that bring meaning to my life?" And then tell your doctor what gives your life meaning.

When it comes to deciding whether a particular surgery or invasive procedure has merit, surgeons are adept at offering statistics. But it's also helpful to push surgeons to tell you what sort of recovery you should expect. Sherwin Nuland tells a story demonstrating that, when it comes to the frail elderly, surgeons may be inclined to underestimate the potholes and length of the postoperative recovery time.

Nuland's ninety-two-year-old patient Hazel Welch was found unconscious by her nursing aides. Nuland suspected that her digestive tract had perforated, which meant that surgery offered her only hope for survival. Once Miss Welch regained her mental faculties, she opined that she had lived long enough. She declined the life-saving operation. But Nuland insisted that she had a one-in-three chance of recovering from surgery, which would be better than certain death. He left her alone to consider her options, and when he returned, she agreed to surgery, stating, "But only because I trust you." Nuland says he suddenly felt less confident that he was doing the right thing.

As any doctor or nurse reading this book will probably guess, the surgery was far more complicated than anticipated. Exploratory surgery in the abdomen can be technically challenging, and the bodies of the extreme elderly pose additional obstacles. It took more than a week to wean Miss Welch from life support and a couple more days before her vocal cords recovered. "When she was able to speak," Nuland says, "she lost no time in letting me know what a dirty trick I had pulled by not letting her die as she wished."

Two weeks after Miss Welch returned to her nursing facility, she suffered a massive stroke and died. Nuland regrets having downplayed potential postoperative difficulties in an attempt to persuade her to go to the operating room. And he wonders whether Miss Welch's ongoing anger at his "well-intentioned deception" helped to trigger the stroke. In retrospect, he says that if he had heeded his own advice, he "would not have been so quick to recommend an operation." Instead, he would have listened to her more and spoken less.

Miss Welch had viewed her abrupt illness as a "gracious way to die," which Nuland had thwarted. But the story serves as a warning to all patients to press their doctors for clarity on the advantages and pitfalls of eleventh-hour treatments or surgeries.

Living Well at the End

At this juncture, I would be remiss for failing to mention a famous study published by a group of doctors from the Massachusetts General Hospital. They looked at patients with diagnoses of metastatic non-small-cell lung cancer—the leading cause of cancer death worldwide. This kind of lung cancer causes much physical suffering, and most people die within a year of diagnosis. This is the same cancer that killed the young neurosurgeon Paul Kalanithi as he was finishing his memoir, *When Breath Becomes Air*. This is also the same cancer with which thirty-four-year-old Sara Monopoli was diagnosed when she was expecting her first child—a story told by the surgeon-writer Atul Gawande.

Non-small-cell lung cancer is a bad cancer, and the doctors at Massachusetts General wanted to see if they could do something to ease the suffering of their patients. So they randomly assigned those with newly diagnosed non-small-cell lung cancer to one of two groups. Half received standard cancer treatment for non-small-cell lung cancer. The other half received standard cancer treatment *plus* early palliative care, which meant that palliative-care doctors and advanced-practice nurses regularly devoted special attention to assessing physical and psychological symptoms, helping with medical decision-making, coordinating care, and establishing patients' medical wishes for the end of life. The palliative-care team provided this assistance throughout the entire course of treatment. By contrast, the first group—the standard treatment group—was not scheduled for such services but could access them upon request.

The results of the study shocked the medical profession. It turns out that early integration of palliative care is extraordinarily effective. But what really shocked doctors was that the patients who received early palliative care lived about two months longer and reported greater quality of life and better moods than those who received standard care. For a disease with a prognosis of less than a year, two additional months of feeling better should not be lightly dismissed.

Even more impressive, however, is that those who received early palliative care opted for less aggressive medical care as they were dying. This meant that they generally received less chemotherapy and more comfort-focused care in the weeks prior to death. What's so remarkable about this is that by opting to focus on quality of life and the preparation for death throughout their treatment for lung cancer, they turned down chemotherapy that was unlikely to help and—compared to those who received standard treatment—enjoyed two more months of life.

In retrospect it might seem obvious that people feel happier when they stay out of the hospital and enjoy life. But what this Massachusetts General study showed is that even when the prognosis is grim and patients are dying, they might live longer when they opt for less aggressive medical care and choose instead to prepare for death.

Every cancer is different, and treatments for advanced diseases differ greatly. The point of the Massachusetts General study is not necessarily that you should forgo life-sustaining therapies or demand palliative care from the moment you receive a dismal diagnosis or poor prognosis—although if palliative care is available, I encourage patients to investigate its resources. Rather, the moral of the story here is that all of us need to engage in the tasks that the palliative-care team facilitated in this study. All of us should acknowledge our finitude and consider carefully—and well before the end—our quality-of-life goals when evaluating treatment options.

Reconsidering Resuscitation

One final aspect of medicalized dying remains to be discussed prior to moving on to some of the other tasks of dying well, and that is the role of cardiopulmonary resuscitation or CPR.

We broached this in Chapter One in the story of Mr. Turner's three deaths and resuscitation attempts. We also touched on it in Chapter Two, with the story of Ms. Capella—my elderly patient with a weak heart, bad lungs, dependence on oxygen, and a dogmatic wish for resuscitation.

Over the course of writing this book, Ms. Capella's memory worsened to the point where she needed around-the-clock care. She remained as feisty as ever, insisting that she wanted all medical interventions possible to keep her alive even a few more hours. But she clearly didn't understand the full implications of this wish.

Her heart already functioned poorly, and were it to stop, she would be dead. We could attempt resuscitation with CPR, but it's hard to jump-start a car with an old faulty engine. Even if you get the motor running again, it'll soon sputter out. The human heart is like that. And if the lungs are no good—as was true for Ms. Capella—there should be no expectation that life support in the form of a mechanical ventilator is going to improve breathing. Life support of this variety is simply maintenance until the next disaster strikes. When the lungs have been irreversibly damaged from a lifetime of smoking or advanced lung cancer, for example, no amount of life support will make a sustained difference.

Today there exists a misguided belief that CPR is uniformly successful and the salve for so much of what ails the human condition. Television and movies no doubt bear some of the blame, because their CPR success rates approach 70 percent. But in the real world, CPR works far less often, and only about

10 to 20 percent of resuscitated patients survive to leave the hospital.

The truth is that most people do not quite realize what CPR entails. The reality is far from the media's tidy portrayal of gentle chest thumps and "mouth-to-mouth." Effective CPR requires rib-fracturing chest compressions. It requires the insertion of a breathing tube and mechanical ventilation of the lungs. It requires large intravenous catheters in major blood vessels for the administration of strong medications to jump-start the heart.

In fact, seriously ill hospitalized patients who have been given the opportunity to learn about CPR are much more likely to decline it. A group of Boston researchers looked at patients over the age of sixty who had less than a year to live. They randomly assigned half of them to watch a three-minute video about heart resuscitation and mechanical ventilation. The other half watched no video. As might be expected, those patients who viewed the video felt better informed about their options. And they were three times as likely to have orders declining CPR than those who did not view the video. Educating patients makes a difference.

Please don't misunderstand. I am a strong proponent of CPR for patients who stand to benefit. As with knee-replacement surgery, CPR is the right intervention for the right person. But in order to identify that "right person," we must take into account frailty, age, lung health, previous open-heart surgeries, and other medical conditions. For some people, CPR imposes far more burden than benefit. Reviving someone who has died comes at a tremendous cost to that person's quality of life. And some patients perceive their new quality of life to be a life worse than death.

Early on in my training, I remember resuscitating a woman in the cardiac intensive-care unit who subsequently told me that she wished we hadn't done it. She was in her late sixties and suffered from difficult-to-control diabetes and heart disease. Unable to manage her weight, she had developed arthritic knees and difficulty walking. This caused her to gain even more weight and eventually to become immobile. She depended on a scooter to get around.

She suffered a massive heart attack and underwent open-heart surgery in our hospital. I met her the day I resuscitated her. When I went back to check on her the next day, she told me she wished we had let her die. I felt defensive.

"But you told us you wanted us to do everything we could to keep you alive," I protested.

"Yes," she replied. "But I changed my mind after going through it." She died again a few weeks later.

Becoming Smaller

My grandmother was ninety-seven years old when I had occasion to visit her in Chicago. Apart from a slow-growing tumor discovered in her stomach a couple of years ago, she was in excellent health. She had no pain and took no medications. Only her memory was a bother. When I went to see her, she had just moved from her own apartment to the memory unit of her complex—a massive building that houses seniors ranging from those who are fully independent to those who are totally dependent.

She was just finishing lunch when I entered, seated in the dining area of the common space, surveying the other residents and staff. Her eyes lit up when she saw me approach, not necessarily because she recognized me, but because she realized that someone was approaching. And I suppose she thought that this someone looked pleasant enough.

"Grandma! It's Lydia! Your granddaughter—Penny's daughter." I introduced myself to the matriarch who had decades earlier rocked me in her arms.

"You're Penny's daughter? Oh how wonderful."

As we chatted, we moved from the common space to her room. I marveled that her whole life had been condensed into one room. As the wife of a bomber pilot turned artist and graphic designer, my grandmother had taken it upon herself to spend money on art. Over the years she had assembled a considerable collection of paintings and sculptures. Her room was decorated with a tasteful sampling, and my uncle had worked hard to re-create the look of her former living room here in the memory unit, much as he had done earlier when she and my grandfather had moved out of their home of fifty-five years into an apartment. Even for me, Grandma's room in the memory unit felt like home—*her* home.

But where had her houseful of possessions gone? The beautiful art? The volumes of family photographs? The hand-crafted furniture? I was vaguely aware that my mother and her siblings had divided some of it up among themselves in an effort to sort through it. Doubtless much got thrown away.

It reminded me of a story I had heard about a woman who held an estate sale as she downsized. Despite hiring a professional company to handle the sale, she made only $2,000. The commission was 50 percent. When she asked the estate sale planner what she should do with the rest of her belongings, he told her that he could haul it all away for $1,000. A lifetime of stuff reduced to nothing.

But there are other less obviously material ways that we become smaller as we age. Our communities shrink. In her prime, my grandmother hosted elaborate dinner parties and entertained my grandfather's business associates, her bridge friends, the neighbors, and her "sewing club" members. Grandma gradually outlived most of her contemporaries, and when my grandfather's health declined prior to her own, she redoubled her commitment to spending her remaining days at his side.

When they first moved out of their home and into the senior complex, I desperately wanted her to make friends. I feared that my grandfather would die, leaving her without a companion. I urged her to invite one of the neighbors over for tea. I promised to do the shopping and prep work for her.

But Grandma had no interest. Her worldly possessions, physical abode, and social connections were shrinking as she herself grew older, smaller, and frailer. It is true that we take nothing with us. And this reality should stir us to consider what *does* matter in the end.

What Matters in the End

It's a good thing to determine what gives our lives meaning—to live on purpose. Studies have shown that having purpose in life is associated with lower rates of cognitive decline and Alzheimer's, less disability, greater happiness, and longer life.

The *New York Times* columnist Paula Span tells the story of her father's longtime friend and neighbor, Manny. A retired kosher butcher, Manny had spent part of his career making home deliveries from his butcher shop. When he reached his nineties, he continued to make house calls, but of a different sort. Daily he checked up on the other elderly residents of his apartment building. Span writes, "Manny was older and frailer than my father; he leaned on a cane and could barely see well enough to recognize faces. But every morning, and again in late afternoon, he walked through my dad's unlocked front door to be sure he was all right and to kibitz a bit. . . . Unless he was ill himself, he never missed a day."

Even as a frail old man, Manny had a clear understanding of what got him out of bed each morning. Although his purpose late in life bore close resemblance to his purpose a half century earlier, it was not precisely the same. It's perfectly reasonable to maintain that what gives our lives meaning can change over time. But the key is to figure out what it is.

I will not attempt to offer a tidy explication of what matters in life, as if there exists some one-size-fits-all approach. But I will say two things on this point. First, determining what ultimately matters requires forethought. Deliberate, considered thinking—not the stuff of mindless daydreaming. Some readers doubtless belong to communities that regularly discuss what gives their lives purpose, but even individuals who inhabit such communities must decide whether to embrace for themselves such corporate beliefs.

Second, determining what matters in the end requires an active response. Let's say, for example, that you have come to believe that family is the most important part of your life. Investing in relationships gives your life meaning, and as you approach retirement, your purpose in life is shifting away from career and toward supporting your grandchildren's well-being and development. The problem is that you live on the other side of the country from your grandchildren, and you only see them a couple of times a year. The determination that investing in family is a core part of your life's purpose may prompt the response of quitting your job and moving closer to family.

If this seems intuitive, it should be. Forty percent of Americans say that spending time with family is the most important source of meaning and fulfillment in their lives, and nearly 70 percent say that time with family gives their lives a "great deal" of meaning. It makes sense that if family is a source of meaning for the majority of Americans, we should adjust our lives in order to prioritize time with family. And if it's not family, but

something else—pursuing a career or perhaps reading philosophy, just to give examples—then we should also determine
how to adjust current life patterns so as to invest more decisively in career or philosophy.

The Pew Research Center recently attempted to figure out
what makes life meaningful for Americans. Researchers took
a two-pronged approach. First, they asked people to use their
own words to describe what gives their lives meaning. People
could say anything they wanted—the question was completely
open-ended. Then the researchers narrowed down responses
to fifteen possible sources of meaning; using these sources they
fashioned a multiple-choice survey.

More than forty-seven hundred people took the two surveys. On the first survey, participants ranked family as the
greatest source of meaning. But after family, the open-ended
responses diverged. A third mentioned career as a source of
meaning, and nearly a quarter cited finances or money. About
one-fifth of respondents indicated that faith and spirituality
provide the most meaning, one-fifth argued for friendships,
and another one-fifth cited various hobbies and activities as the
greatest source of fulfillment. There you have it: family, work,
and money score highest for offering meaning to American
lives. And spirituality, friendships, and activities tie for fourth.

On the multiple-choice survey, however, when asked to
identify the single most important source of meaning for their
lives, 20 percent of Americans chose religion, second only to
family.

Should this data do anything for us? Perhaps it's reassuring—

our priorities align with those of others. But perhaps it's revealing—we've never given much thought to the sources of meaning and fulfillment for our lives. Or if we have, we've not bothered to change anything to support the realization of our priorities.

If my grandmother had taken the Pew surveys, she would in no way have been a statistical outlier. God and family had always topped her list. And she oriented her life in such a way as to realize these priorities. Weekly church attendance, for example, was a must. And she was as loyal as they come to family. Her husband, my grandfather, was not the easiest life partner. Although Grandma once scooped up their three small children and left him for a time, she ultimately stuck with their marriage. She told me later, "If it took fifty years for your grandfather to become the man he became, it was worth the wait."

Over her lifetime, Grandma cultivated disciplines and virtues that enabled her not only to endure a tough marriage but also to flourish. She flourished personally, saw to the flourishing of her family, and eventually experienced a flourishing marriage. My grandfather died in 2016, just two months after celebrating their seventieth wedding anniversary.

Flourishing While Dying

If the art of dying well is in truth the art of living well, then how ought we to live? How might we face death and still flourish? The ancient Greek philosophers Plato and Aristotle thought that if you wanted to do anything well, you had—at the very least—to live a life of virtue.

If a "life of virtue" sounds like a turnoff, hear me out. The Greeks understood the virtues to be excellent habits that a person could cultivate over a lifetime. If you were lucky, Aristotle taught, you were born into a good family that cared about how you were shaped as a human being. As a child you learned such virtues as courage, justice, and self-control. These didn't necessarily come naturally, but you worked at them. And with a lot of practice and the practical wisdom that comes with age, you could attain a virtuous or excellent life that would make your flourishing possible. In other words, the cultivation of good habits and practices within the context of social relationships leads to human flourishing.

But is it possible to flourish while dying? Aristotle would have said that it isn't. For Aristotle, a person also needed external goods like health, wealth, and friends to be able to flourish. But Plato and the ancient Stoics believed that virtue was sufficient. According to their logic, someone who had cultivated the habits of excellence could in fact flourish while dying.

As I was completing this book, my grandmother was in decline. When I visited her in the memory unit, she appeared thinner than ever. Although she had no pain, my suspicion was that the tumor in her stomach was growing. It was deemed "inoperable" two years ago when it was discovered—both because of her frailty and because of the extent of its spread. There was no question that Grandma was dying. Yet she flourished, exuding serenity and grace even as her world grew smaller.

This book is filled with stories of people who flourished in their dying. What, then, is the secret? What excellences should we cultivate throughout our lives in order to die well—in order to reinvigorate the art of dying today?

If we adopt Susan Sontag's notion of illness as metaphor, we might propose developing the virtue of courage in our attempt to vanquish that feared enemy death. But, as I previously suggested, trying to conquer fear of death may be the wrong project. Rather, we are to persist in walking with those we love toward the fear and sadness—a harrowing, noble task.

Others might propose that we concentrate on the much-heralded Western virtue of self-determination. If anything defines America, this may be it. Pioneers and explorers going it alone, forging their own paths. At first blush, we might think rugged individualism a useful excellence for succeeding at anything, including dying well. But Aristotle was correct when he said that no one flourishes in isolation. As spelled out earlier, we are relational beings, and dying is a community affair. It takes a village to flourish while dying.

There are other virtues—ancient and modern—around which we could attempt to create some sort of guide to dying well. Perhaps justice. Perhaps love. These do indeed have merit in and of themselves, yet it strikes me as arbitrary to elect them over any others. So we return to our question about what virtues we must cultivate in order to die well, and our inability to answer this forces us to reconsider the original *ars moriendi*, which had a very decisive description of what it takes to die well. What habits did the *ars moriendi* suggest?

Recall the illustrated *Ars moriendi*, which paired five temptations commonly faced by the dying with five virtues that mitigate the temptations. Remember the image of the dying man, impatient with his slow decline, anxious to get on with death? Impatience, the *ars moriendi* taught, can be moderated through the lifelong cultivation of the virtue of patience. The transformation does not happen instantly when a person wills it. Patience must be practiced. Like any habit, you have to commit to exercising patience over and over and over again.

So too with the other virtues that the *ars moriendi* commended the dying to cultivate. The tendency to despair as death approaches can be remedied through a lifetime of exercising hopefulness. The arrogant and self-absorbed might practice humility—a welcoming and inclusive virtue. Those tempted to doubt their religious convictions might find strength through a life of nurturing their faith. And finally, those who cling most stringently to the material goods of this world can mitigate such avarice through the practice of generosity. In fact, since you can't take it with you and your world will shrink one day anyway, start the habit now of giving your stuff away.

In the end, these virtues—patience, hope, humility, faith, and "letting go"—lead to flourishing through life as through death. In reflecting on the themes of this book, the habit of letting go makes possible the acknowledgment of human finitude, and the habit of humility makes space for community—recognizing finitude and embracing community being the foundational elements of an art of dying. Exercising faith together with hope helps to mitigate fear of death, suggests answers to our deepest existential anxieties, and promotes the cultivation of peace. And nearly all of us could do with more patience—every day of our living and our dying.

But one should not wait to begin cultivating these virtues.

The mid-twentieth-century chaplain of the United States Senate, Peter Marshall, might best be known for his telling of the legend of the merchant of Baghdad. The story goes like this.

A merchant sends his servant down to the market. The servant quickly returns. He is agitated and frightened. He says to his master, "Down at the marketplace I was jostled by a woman in the crowd, and when I turned around I saw it was Death that jostled me. She looked at me and made a threatening gesture. Master, please lend me your horse, for I must hasten away to avoid her. I will ride to Samarra and there I will hide, and Death will not find me."

The merchant agrees, lends his horse, and the servant wastes no time in galloping off. Later that day, the merchant himself heads down to the market and finds Death standing in the crowd. He asks her why she made a threatening gesture at his servant that morning.

Death replies, "That was not a threatening gesture. It was only a start of surprise. I was astonished to see him in Baghdad, for I have an appointment with him tonight in Samarra."

This story reminds us that none of us escapes our appointment with death. The solution is neither to flee it nor to seek it out. Rather, we must each prepare for Samarra. Death is part of life. The art of dying well must necessarily be wrapped up in the art of living.

On Beauty Lost

For each person, there is a point at which the art of dying begins to outpace the art of living. For my grandmother, this occurred shortly before I left for a work trip. Her hospice nurse, Donna, texted to say that Grandma had rolled out of bed. Donna believed that my grandmother was showing signs of "terminal agitation"—a burst of restlessness displayed by the actively dying. She asked my thoughts on prescribing sedatives. By the time we had finished our exchange, however, the staff had settled Grandma in a recliner in the common area, within their view. We agreed to give sedation only if absolutely necessary.

The next day I was to speak at a conference on the opioid crisis. Donna texted again to report that my grandmother had become unresponsive and was breathing quickly. "I need to give morphine for breathing and pain," she wrote. Although an appropriate suggestion, it struck me as odd to discuss giving morphine during a conference on opiates.

The truth is that morphine and its sister drugs, when taken at the end of life, do not contribute to the opioid crisis. They are often used to relieve pain and to calm the labored breathing of the dying. Because these medications can also make the dying process appear more serene by masking involuntary grimaces and gasps, they are sometimes used even when pa-tients aren't in pain or experiencing difficulty breathing. In my grandmother's case, she showed no evidence of pain and her breathing was rapid but not labored, so we opted to hold the morphine.

A year earlier my grandmother had been unresponsive for several days. We were told that death was imminent and began to make funeral arrangements. Grandma was so lethargic that her nurses stopped administering her painkillers. After several days, she woke up, and everyone realized that she was not dy-ing at all. Rather, she had unwittingly been given too many opiates.

The day after the opioid conference, I was to speak at an-other conference on the topic of responses to human suffering. My phone buzzed during the plenary session with a text from Donna. "Just got the call that she passed away. I'm calling Pam now"—no final punctuation to her text.

My grandmother had been largely unresponsive for a cou-ple of days. The preceding night, her children and some ex-tended family had gathered at her bedside with her pastor. In true *ars moriendi* fashion, they sang, prayed, and shared stories. Grandma's eyes had been closed throughout, but she squeezed the pastor's hand as if to signal her gratitude that the group had assembled. The evening brought great closure for everyone. The next afternoon, she fell asleep, never to awake.

I slipped out of the plenary session and called my mother. She had just arrived at the lobby of my grandmother's building, still unaware that she had been orphaned not minutes before. Donna and I had both tried to reach my aunt, but without success. Then I phoned my uncle. He was on his way home from work, planning to head over to my grandmother's.

There followed texts and phone calls to siblings and cousins. Reflections. Kind words. Not a single person could muster a hint of negativity or sarcasm for our graceful Grandma.

Suddenly the finality of her nearly ninety-eight years overwhelmed me. I stepped outside, planted myself on a bench in the sun, and started to cry.

I should have been able to rationalize it. I had seen so much death, and we had known for years now that Grandma carried cancerous masses in her stomach and liver. In the last couple of weeks she had lost a lot of weight and had hardly risen from bed. I had spent the last thirty-six hours intensely coordinating her care and translating the signs of dying for my family.

But grief overpowers rationality, and I wept. I wept not for her death. Grandma indeed had lived an incredibly long and healthy life. Her dying had been painless and peaceful. I did not weep because I no longer had a grandparent. Nor even because I hadn't been there at the end.

Rather, I lamented the loss of the gentlest woman I had ever known. Wise and kind and selfless. A woman whose faith had sustained her through poverty and war and a half century of a difficult marriage. A woman who prayed daily for the flourishing of her children, grandchildren, and great-grandchildren.

She brought beauty to the world by virtue of her being in the world. And with her death, the world lost some of its beauty. An annual—not a perennial—gently plucked from the earth, never to blossom here again.

During the days immediately following Grandma's death, I found myself wishing that I could clothe myself in traditional mourning attire so that I didn't have to explain to colleagues and strangers the reason for my sadness. I wished I didn't have to go to the office or take care of patients. In my distress, the significance of mourning rituals became all the more real to me, and I yearned for the freedom that such practices provide. But modern life—and especially the practice of modern medicine—rarely makes space for grief. Since I couldn't take a physical leave from work, I gave myself a mental *shivah*, a seven-day space to sit low and mourn.

I wondered anew how equipped we who have lost the *ars moriendi* are to handle the sorrow of beauty lost.

On Taking a Breath Together

Could Mr. Turner have died better if he had lived differently? Would he have been resuscitated three times? This book doubtless makes all of us reflect on deaths we've experienced. We second-guess the decisions we've made. "I wish Dad could have died at home," or, "Maybe we should have stopped chemo sooner." But the aim of this book is not to induce regret but to provide the substance for change moving forward.

It's meant to compel us to think differently about our *living*—
and thereby to improve our dying.

One of the most extraordinary events I have witnessed as
a physician is the time a music therapist visited an elderly patient with advanced dementia. She could not get out of bed,
rarely opened her eyes, and had to be spoon-fed. She never,
ever spoke. Family members told the therapist, a violinist, that
"Amazing Grace" had been one of the woman's favorite songs.
As the violin released the notes of that quiet, hopeful melody,
the old woman opened her mouth and began to sing, her voice
cracking yet steady, mostly on pitch. She could no longer talk.
But she could sing.

Those who care for patients with advanced dementia know
for a fact that singing is one of the last remaining ways that
people with advanced Alzheimer's can participate in the life
of a community—and experience beauty.

Elaine Stratton Hild is a musicologist with an interest in
medieval chants for the sick and dying. She came to the field,
in part, because her own career as an accomplished violist was
cut short by a debilitating neurologic disease. But while she
could still play, as a student at Cleveland Institute of Music,
Hild had the opportunity to play for patients in hospitals and
hospices. She experienced firsthand the ritual use of music—
creating order from chaos—and she saw how music tightens
the bonds of community.

"When a group of people sing together, they have to
breathe together," Hild says. "When we're losing a loved one,
sometimes it's hard to breathe. Yet the community is forced

to take a breath together, and to match their breath and their voices to one another. It joins the community together, and it's something beautiful to do for someone who's just gone beyond your reach."

Art enables us to experience beauty in community as our bodies decay without our permission. Music provides the substance around which we blend our voices—and our exhalations.

Last Words

Since the beginning, poets and philosophers, sculptors and painters, writers and readers alike have found death an unseemly inspiration. Death can be as profound as a bottomless well and as unrestrained as a starving lion. It at once baffles and consumes us.

The *ars moriendi* sought to tame death. Throughout this book, we have considered many of the ways it did so. But we have not yet discussed one aspect of the "art of dying"—the last words of the dying.

One of the earliest literary records of last words is attributed to the Hebrew patriarch Jacob. Just before he died, Jacob gathered his twelve sons and pronounced on each an individual blessing. To his son Reuben, he said, "You are my firstborn, . . . excelling in rank and excelling in power." He declared of his youngest: "Benjamin is a ravenous wolf, in the morning devouring the prey, and at evening dividing the spoil." These last

words left no doubt in each son's mind how their father understood them and how they were to live out the rest of their lives.

Jacob then issued instructions for his final rest. He wished
to be buried in the cave where his parents and grandparents
were buried, in a distant land. He spared no detail in describing his wishes and had his son Joseph swear an oath that he
would follow his orders. The story tells us that, having finished
his business, Jacob died.

If the *ars moriendi* tradition made much of last words, it
was the Methodists who championed them. Methodism arose
in the eighteenth century as a revival movement within the
Church of England. Its followers believed firmly that life is a
rehearsal for death—living well is necessary for dying well—
and the hour of death provided the opportunity to confirm
the authenticity of belief. As the scholar Shai Lavi puts it, "Dying was not merely another event in the life of the Methodist;
it was the culminating moment through which the entirety of
life could be understood."

The Methodists took to recording the last hours of life in
what they called "biographies." These differed from what we
think of as obituaries today. The biographies focused not on
the dead person's lifetime achievements, but almost exclu-
sively on the dying process itself. How did the believer act?
What did he or she say? What were the last words? Witnesses
described deathbed scenes in detail and published them in
regional journals. Community members studied them carefully as examples of how to die well. Although such scripts for
dying eventually lost their influence, people everywhere have

continued to pay attention to what a person says just before death.

Indeed, last words take many forms. They may, as with Jacob, bless or instruct. Last words might be issued as apologies or requests for forgiveness. Leonardo da Vinci's last words expressed humility and regret; he lamented that he had offended God and his fellow human beings because—believe it or not—the quality of his work had been insufficient. Some people assure those gathered of their love and affection. Still others may describe the liminal—that mystical threshold between life and whatever awaits. Thomas Edison, long considered America's greatest inventor, fell into a coma during his last days. Just before he died he returned to consciousness. Looking up, he said, "It is very beautiful over there." Apple cofounder Steve Jobs said simply, "Oh wow. Oh wow. Oh wow."

Many writers feel that a book's opening sentence is its most important. But if a person's life represents a story, it is often the final chapter—the concluding sentences—that leave the largest impact.

I began this book by saying that I regretted that we resuscitated Mr. W. J. Turner. He didn't have to die as he did. And I hold him up as an example of how we must all take the opportunity to anticipate our mortality and prepare for death—engaging our families, our communities, and our medical teams in the effort. The art of dying is really the art of living.

The body withers and fades—this is surely to be expected. But we are not without resources—existential, ritual, practical. And as we walk together toward the fear and the sadness, as we sit low to grieve our own dying or the death of others, we may find ourselves transformed in the process. The transformation is not from sickness to health or from death to life. Rather, it is the change that comes from experiencing the profound. We grow wiser, more whole. We discover calm in turmoil, light in shadow, beauty in decay.

Art for a New *Ars Moriendi*,
by Michael W. Dugger

This is a book on the *art* of dying. By this point, you've read narrative, essay, poetry, philosophy, and theology. You've read about music. You've read about the Isenheim altarpiece. And you've read that one of the earliest versions of the *Ars moriendi* was illustrated, enabling all who encountered it—not least the illiterate and uneducated—to reflect on their finitude and prepare for death.

There is a way in which art stirs us to moral action. Beauty provokes desire, to be sure, but art can also prompt other responses. In the case of the *ars moriendi*, the art of human finitude provokes anticipation and preparation for an inevitable end.

Early on in the writing of this book, a colleague challenged me to consider whether it would be possible to reclaim a visual practice to accompany my narrative. Could text alone do justice to the *art* of dying? My colleague argued that the book would be more engaging if each chapter were paired with an image.

To this end, I commissioned the artist Michael W. Dugger—whose own work engages with fundamentally existential questions—to create ink renderings in response to the original *ars moriendi* woodcuts. The goal was to design a modern image that could also develop the themes of each chapter. In what follows, you will find the fruits of this labor: an image for each chapter paired with its description.

ONE

DEATH

This is Mr. W. J. Turner, the elderly African American gentleman whom I describe at the book's outset. As a *moriens,* or dying man, this is also the image that most closely approximates the original *ars moriendi* woodcuts reproduced in Chapter Two.

Several elements make this image distinct from those of the fifteenth century. One is Mr. Turner's African ancestry. Another is the presence of modern hospital equipment in a modern hospital room. What's more, the image lacks any sort of intrinsic morality. If the *ars moriendi* illustrations paired temptations with consolations for the dying, this image tells the story of a death that occurs in a hospital, devoid of any larger narrative. This is precisely the story that this book seeks to disrupt.

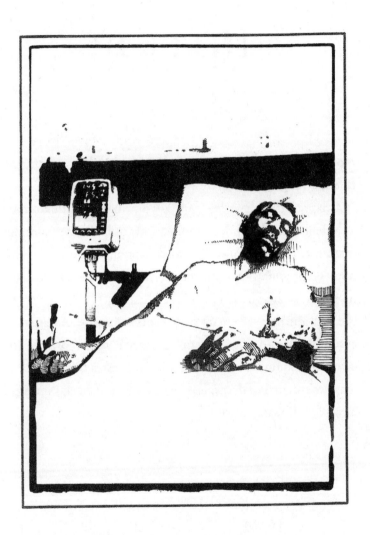

TWO

FINITUDE

Flowers represent the idea of the temporal and the temporary. By their very nature, cut flowers endure only briefly.

Chapter Two describes *vanitas* paintings—art that served as a deliberate reminder of human finitude. These paintings often incorporated flowers into their compositions. For this book's representation of the finite, the artist chose the lily. The flower illustrated here remains attached to its bulb, suggesting the "life journey" of a plant from roots to flowers. A perennial evokes more enduring patterns of time. Furthermore, the lily is a common funeral flower: its scent possesses the strength to mask the stench of decay. It is also an Easter flower, hinting at new life following death.

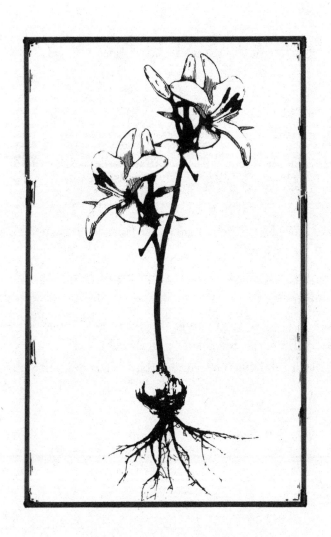

THREE

COMMUNITY

This chapter opens with two juxtaposed stories of lonely dying—in America and Japan.

This image evokes the *danchi,* the stacked Japanese apartment complexes where many older Japanese are experiencing lonely deaths. The top frame of this two-part image shows Mrs. Ito, the isolated elderly woman in her apartment. Her open paper screen, relic of an older way of living, suggests that she is still alive. The bottom frame shows the screen mostly closed. The text is the Japanese for "lonely death."

The art of dying is best understood as a community affair.

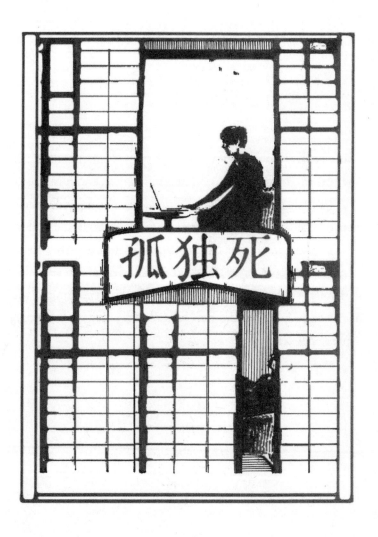

FOUR

CONTEXT

This chapter explores why the majority of Americans die in institutions, such as hospitals, nursing homes, and hospices.

A gentleman in a wheelchair provides a visual representation of the many people who grow increasingly dependent on the mechanisms of health-care institutions. This rising reliance on doctors and hospitals—both individually and societally—is partly responsible for the fact that only a minority of people die at home, contradicting their own strongly expressed wishes.

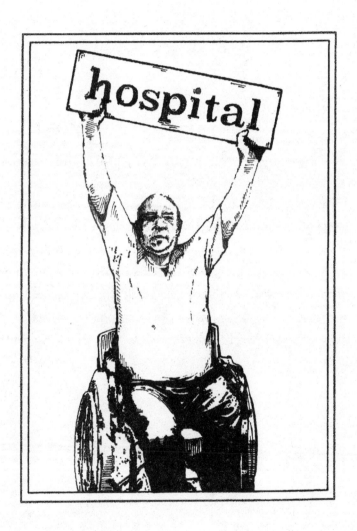

FIVE

FEAR

For a chapter on fear, this image was designed to represent—as well as to induce—its subject.

This is a disturbing piece of art, and over the course of its many renditions the artist toned it down significantly. A young woman, eyes wide open in terror, lies in a hospital bed that bears a striking resemblance to an open coffin. It is not exactly clear whether the oxygen mask is helping or smothering her. Her arms are hidden, which prompts the viewer to ask whether she has the ability to escape from the encroaching darkness.

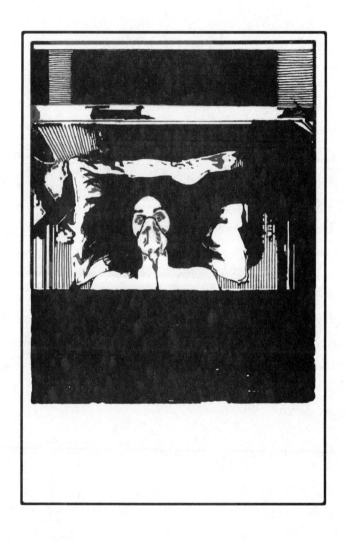

SIX

BODY

This image is also disquieting. If we reject the idea of contemplating our finitude, we must also reject the idea that our bodies will, one day, fail.

The figure is an erect, humanized form of the hybrid creature from the Isenheim Altarpiece described in the chapter's text—as Huysmans puts it, his "legs spread wide, bloated belly pushing against the surrounding darkness. His skin is littered with the haloed lesions of St. Anthony's Fire." If compared to the creature in the altarpiece painting, the viewer will soon observe the similarities. The aim is to prompt a visual reckoning with bodily finitude while also noting that disease can transfigure even as it transforms.

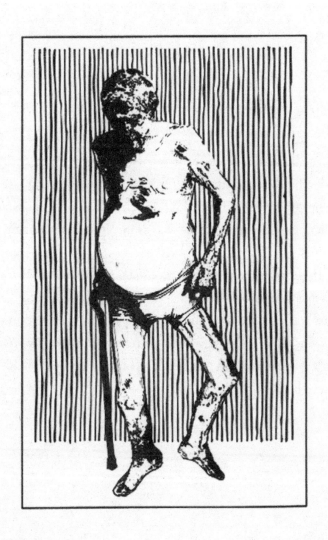

SEVEN

SPIRIT

For a discussion of spirit, it seemed appropriate to present stained glass as another art form closely related to an art of dying. Stained glass can be found in churches, synagogues, and other houses of worship, as well as in cemeteries and funeral parlors.

This image links the notion of *shalom* (written in Hebrew) to what is described in the chapter as "vandalized shalom." The glass is composed of fragments, more clearly shattered in the bottom half. The dove, which represents peace or *shalom,* is itself fragmented and inverted. Preparation for death helps to rescue us from vandalized *shalom.*

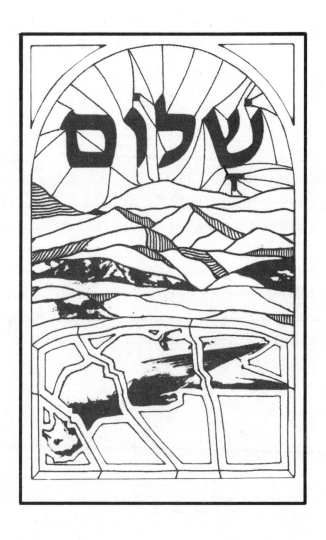

EIGHT

RITUAL

The image of a burial draws together many Western death-related rituals, including those performed in the hospital prior to death, preparing a body for burial, and funerary rituals.

In this image, a group of men lowers a coffin into the ground; but the space where the hole should be is empty. The suspension of the coffin in space—indeed the realization that the men themselves are suspended—underscores the existential and emotional chaos brought about by death. Ritual creates order in the midst of such chaos.

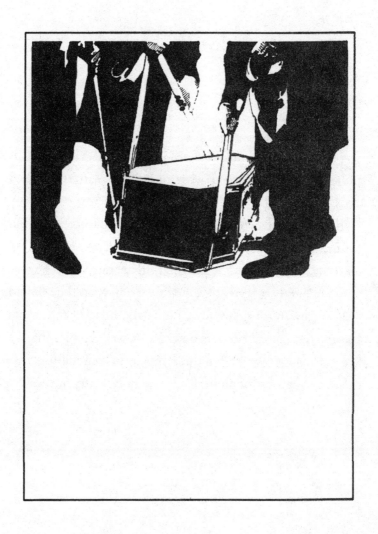

NINE

LIFE

The themes of the book coalesce in this final chapter, which addresses questions about what ultimately matters for each of us.

This image of a young boy with his grandmother exemplifies the answer that most people give when asked what brings meaning to their lives. For a chapter titled "Life," the representation of family suggests that the threat of our finitude should drive us toward those we love. But it also highlights how life continues despite death's shadow. To die well requires that we live well, and we live best in the company of communities that help us make sense of our finitude and find beauty in decay.

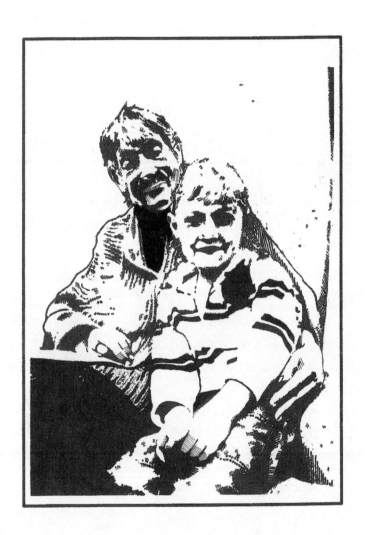

AUTHOR'S NOTE

I am grateful to both colleagues and patients for their part-
nership over the years. To protect the privacy of both, I
have changed names and identifying details. When my memory has failed me or I wished to illustrate a point more vividly,
I have re-created or combined elements of patients' stories.

There are several exceptions, however. My patient Diana
Atwood Johnson gave me permission to write explicitly about
her life and death. Diana died on January 1, 2018. Jill Pellett
Levine agreed to let me tell the story of the death of her husband, Jesse Levine, in 2008. And I share the story of my grandmother's death as I experienced it.

With regard to endnotes, I have omitted superscript numbers from the text. If you wish to see references for works or
studies cited, the notes section at the end of the book lists
them by page number and key words in the order that they
appear throughout the book.

WITH GRATITUDE

I owe heartfelt thanks to the many friends who supported me as I wrote this book. I started writing while on faculty at Yale School of Medicine and finished as a faculty member of Columbia University. I have been encouraged by more people than I can possibly name.

I am especially grateful, however, to Philip Laughlin, who prompted me to propose this book, and to Barry Nalebuff, who pushed me to dream big. Barry introduced me to my wonderful agent, Susan Ginsburg, who has advocated for me tirelessly.

I am grateful to Patrick Hough and the Elm Institute for supporting my writing. I thank Yale's Griswold Fund for underwriting my research trip to Colmar, France. And I thank my dear friend Ted Snyder for helping to commission the artwork for this book.

I am indebted to friends at Veritas for providing the occasion for me to meet my editor. I owe my biggest debt to the unassuming, ever wise Francis Su. Francis knows why.

My editor, Mickey Maudlin, has been a constant source of wisdom. I am grateful that he took a chance on me and tolerated my countless "clipped and confident" emails.

Friends, colleagues, professors, and patients have provided stories and inspiration, have advised on the manuscript, or have permitted me to work out my ideas in conversation. My sincere thanks to Awet Andemicael, Teresa Berger, Daniel Callahan, Matt Coburn, Drew Collins, Leo Cooney, Eric Dugdale, Lucinda Dugger, Michael W. Dugger, Richard Egan, Eliana Falk, Greg Ganssle, Janie Ghazarossian, William Goettler, John Hare, Mark Heim, Jennifer Herdt, Anita Hinkson, Jon Hinkson, Kyle Humphrey, Jill Pellett Levine, Christian Lundberg, Edith Newfield, Tracy Rabin, Markus Rathey, Marjorie Rosenthal, Jane Salk, Nicole Shirilla, Linnéa Spransy, Peter Wicks, Christian Wiman, and Miroslav Wolf. I thank my friends Rebecca McLaughlin and Tanya Walker, who read and commented on the manuscript. I'm also grateful to my husband, Kyle, who scrutinized every word at least once.

Care of the dying requires a team, and I thank those who cared for my patient Diana at the end, including Elaine Bonoan, Danielle Antin-Ozerkis, the medical ICU staff, and Diana's rich community of friends and family. I am also immensely grateful to those who attended my grandmother during her final days, especially her hospice nurse, Donna, and her children, Pamella Christensen, Penelope Stickney, and Kurt Ulrich.

After my grandmother's funeral, my family and I gathered around a table in the restaurant of the hotel where we were staying. Conversation turned to this book and its accompanying artwork—still a work in progress at the time. Michael pulled up preparatory sketches of the images on his phone and passed them around, and we deliberated over their symbolism. Faith and family matter for me—as they did for my grandmother—and evenings such as that one make me especially grateful. A mere thanks hardly suffices for my parents, Phil and Penny, for my siblings, Luke, Lucinda, and Leah, and their families, or for Kyle and our daughters, Eloise and Susannah. Thankfully, these are not my last words.

Chapter 1: Death

6 *A recent Harvard study found . . . :* T. A. Balboni et al., "Provision of
Spiritual Support to Patients with Advanced Cancer by Religious
Communities and Associations with Medical Care at the End of Life,"
JAMA Internal Medicine 173/12 (2013): 1109–17 (1113).

7 *Recognizing that such patients . . . :* J. J. Sanders et al., "Seeking and
Accepting: U.S. Clergy Theological and Moral Perspectives Informing
Decision Making at the End of Life," *Journal of Palliative Medicine*
20/10 (October 2017): 1059–67.

8 *The Harvard study found . . . :* Balboni et al., "Provision of Spiritual
Support."

13 *One doctor describes hospitals as . . . :* Steven Swinford and Laura Hughes,
"Hospitals Act like 'Conveyor Belts' for Dying Patients," *The Telegraph*,
August 13, 2015, http://www.telegraph.co.uk/news/nhs/11802113
/Hospitals-act-like-conveyor-belts-for-dying-patients.html.

13 *invoking the so-called* dis*assembly lines . . . :* Swift & Company's Meat
Packing House, Chicago, Illinois, "Splitting Backbones and Final
Inspection of Hogs," 1910–1915, https://www.thehenryford.org
/collections-and-research/digital-collections/artifact/354536.

13 *"The idea is that a man must not . . .":* Henry Ford, *My Life and Work*,
1922 (CreateSpace, 2017), 41.

16 *My grandfather Norman Ulrich . . . :* I have published my grandfather's story elsewhere. See Lydia Dugdale, "Healing the Dying," *First Things*, December 2016, 45–49.

18 *He went on to publish* The Decameron . . . : Giovanni Boccaccio, *The Decameron*, trans. Wayne A. Rebhorn (New York: Norton, 2014), 6.

19 *"writhing about as if . . .":* Boccaccio, *Decameron*, 7.

19 *"to fortify the brain . . . against the stinking air . . .":* Boccaccio, *Decameron*, 8.

19 *"The number of people dying . . .":* Boccaccio, *Decameron*, 9.

19 *Historians estimate that as much as . . . :* Lydia Dugdale, "The Art of Dying Well," *Hastings Center Report* 40/6 (2010): 22–24.

20 *"The stench of their decaying bodies . . .":* Boccaccio, *Decameron*, 11.

Chapter 2: Finitude

28 *Worldwide average life expectancy increased . . . :* World Bank, "Life Expectancy at Birth, Total (Years)," https://data.worldbank.org /indicator/SP.DYN.LE00.IN?end=2015&start=1960&view=chart.

28 *In 1960, 12.2 percent of babies worldwide . . . :* World Bank, "Mortality Rate, Infant (per 1,000 Live Births)," https://data.worldbank.org /indicator/SP.DYN.IMRT.IN?end=2017&start=1960&view=chart.

30 *Accounts of these "triumphs" vary . . . :* Mary Beard, *The Roman Triumph* (Cambridge, MA: Harvard Univ. Press, 2009), 85–92.

30 *Socrates taught that the principal goal . . . :* See Plato's *Phaedo*, in *Plato: Complete Works,* ed. J. M. Cooper (Indianapolis: Hackett, 1997), 64a.

31 *Qohelet, the "Teacher" of Hebrew scripture . . . :* Eccles. 12:1, 7 (NRSV).

31 *One genre of art related . . . :* Eccles. 1:2 (NRSV).

31 *Compared with the infinite, the logic goes . . . :* Eccles. 3:20.

34 *The work explained in concrete terms . . . :* For example, the work drew slightly from earlier liturgical material by Friar Laurent, Henry Suso, and Dirk van Delft.

34 *Gerson's handbook was meant for . . . :* Sister Mary Catharine O'Connor, *The Art of Dying Well: The Development of the Ars Moriendi* (New York: Columbia Univ. Press, 1942), 23. This is the first comprehensive American academic work on the *ars moriendi*.

34 *It became popular . . . :* O'Connor, *Art of Dying Well*, 23.

34 *In 1415, an anonymous author . . . :* In addition to Gerson's influence, the *Tractatus* draws from Stoic thought, patristic writings, and Catholic liturgy.

34 *Its title is considered . . . :* My overview of the *ars moriendi* here owes substantial credit to O'Connor, *Art of Dying Well*, 1–45; and Allen

Verhey, *The Christian Art of Dying: Learning from Jesus* (Grand Rapids, MI: Eerdmans, 2011), 79–88.

35 *The* ars moriendi *ignored . . . :* David William Atkinson, *The English Ars Moriendi*, Renaissance and Baroque Studies and Texts, vol. 5 (New York: Peter Lang, 1992), 1.

35 *"to die well is to die gladly and willfully":* In the Old English: "to dye wele ys to dye gladely and wylfully" (Atkinson, *English* Ars Moriendi, 2).

36 *Consumers of the* ars moriendi *texts . . . :* Although Gerson does not mention these temptations in his *Scientia mortis*, their description came to be regarded as the most important aspect of the *ars moriendi*, perhaps because they relate directly to the experience of the dying.

37 *"makes it quite clear . . .":* O'Connor, *Art of Dying Well*, 5–6.

37 *"a complete and intelligible guide . . .":* O'Connor, *Art of Dying Well*, 5.

41 *western Europe required access . . . :* Antony Griffiths, *Prints and Printmaking: An Introduction to the History and Techniques* (London: British Museum Press, 2010), 16. John Harthan, in *The History of the Illustrated Book* (London: Thames and Hudson, 1981), generally agrees with Griffiths's analysis, although he does point out that a well-known woodcut block print of St. Christopher is dated 1423, and it is unclear whether this date refers to the year in which the woodcut was carved or in which the impression was made.

41 *Advice on dying well appeared in health manuals . . . :* See Lydia S. Dugdale, "Desecularizing Death," *Christian Bioethics* 23/1 (2017): 22–37.

42 *"By the 1860s many elements of the Good Death . . .":* Drew Gilpin Faust, *This Republic of Suffering: Death and the American Civil War* (New York: Vintage, 2008), 7.

44 *At random times of day and night . . . :* See https://www.wecroak.com. Also see Bianca Bosker, "The App That Reminds You You're Going to Die: It Helped Me Find Inner Peace," *Atlantic*, January/February 2018, https://www.theatlantic.com/magazine/archive/2018/01/when-death-pings/546587.

Chapter 3: Community

48 *The journalist N. R. Kleinfield's . . . :* N. R. Kleinfield, "The Lonely Death of George Bell," *New York Times*, October 17, 2015, https://www.nytimes.com/2015/10/18/nyregion/dying-alone-in-new-york-city.html.

50 *"A Generation in Japan . . .":* Norimitsu Onishi, "A Generation in Japan Faces a Lonely Death," *New York Times*, November 30, 2017.

50 *"We are fools to depend upon . . .":* Blaise Pascal, *Pensées*, trans. W. F. Trotter (New York: Dutton, 1958), 61–62.

52 *In fact, Ariès reports . . . :* Philippe Ariès, *The Hour of Our Death*, 2nd ed., trans. Helen Weaver (New York: Vintage, 2008), 19.

54 *"She summoned all her servants . . .":* This account of Madame de Montespan is taken from Ariès, *Hour of Our Death,* 18–19, which is based on Louis de Rouvroy duc de Saint-Simon, *Mémoires* (Paris: Les Grands Ecrivains de la France, 1901), 15: 486.

61 *The palliative-care doctor Ira Byock . . . :* Ira Byock, *Dying Well: Peace and Possibilities at the End of Life* (New York: Riverhead, 1997), 275.

61 *Byock notes that hospice . . . :* Byock, *Dying Well,* 140.

62 *"I'm dying. I know I'm dying . . .":* Lydia Dugdale, *Dying in the Twenty-First Century: Toward a New Ethical Framework for the Art of Dying Well* (Cambridge, MA: MIT Press, 2015), 173.

62 *"consider its excesses in light of . . .":* Dugdale, *Dying in the Twenty-First Century,* 174.

62 *"Community helps us to recognize . . .":* Dugdale, *Dying in the Twenty-First Century,* 174.

69 *"Death was always public":* Ariès, *Hour of Our Death,* 19.

Chapter 4: Context

72 *Indeed, some 80 percent of Americans . . . :* Stanford School of Medicine, Palliative Care, "Home Care of the Dying Patient: Where Do Americans Die?" https://palliative.stanford.edu/home-hospice-home-care-of-the-dying-patient/where-do-americans-die.

72 *Although the average American moves . . . :* Mona Chalabi, "How Many Times Does the Average Person Move?" *FiveThirtyEight*, January 29, 2015, https://fivethirtyeight.com/features/how-many-times-the-average-person-moves.

74 *Heidegger describes . . . :* Martin Heidegger, *Poetry, Language, Thought,* trans. Albert Hofstadter (New York: Harper & Row, 1971), 157–58.

75 *Why does only one in five Americans . . . :* Stanford School of Medicine, "Home Care of the Dying Patient."

75 *Basil of Caesarea, a fourth-century . . . :* Thomas Heyne, "Reconstructing the World's First Hospital: The Basiliad," *Hektoen International*, Spring 2015.

75 *In Philippe Ariès's collection . . . :* Philippe Ariès, *The Hour of Our Death*, 2nd ed., trans. Helen Weaver (New York: Vintage, 2008), 570.

76 *Starr describes the family . . . :* Paul Starr, *The Social Transformation of American Medicine: The Rise of a Sovereign Profession and the Making of a Vast Industry,* 2nd ed. (New York: Basic Books, 2017), 32.

77 *Buchan's book remained popular . . . :* Starr, *Social Transformation,* 32–33.

77 *They were to become beacons of hope . . . :* Starr, *Social Transformation,* 145.

78 *"What drove this transformation . . .":* Starr, *Social Transformation,* 146.

78 *"a workplace for the production of health":* Starr, *Social Transformation,* 146.

79 *In 1873, there existed fewer than . . . :* Starr, *Social Transformation,* 73.

80 *"Our moral response to the imminence of death . . .":* Albert R. Jonsen, "Bentham in a Box: Technology Assessment and Heath Care Allocation," *Law, Medicine, and Health Care* 14/3–4 (1986): 174.

81 *"rescue fantasy is a power trip . . .":* Howard Brody, *The Healer's Power* (New Haven, CT: Yale Univ. Press, 1992), 139.

82 *"I was speechless when she gave it back . . .":* Marjorie S. Rosenthal, "Caregiver-Centered Care," *Journal of the American Medical Association* 311/10 (March 12, 2014): 1015.

82 *Later, Rosenthal reminded him . . . :* Marjorie S. Rosenthal, "Why We Need to Talk About Alzheimer's," *Time,* November 23, 2015, http://time.com/4119648/national-alzheimers-disease-and-caregiver-month.

83 *More than sixteen million Americans . . . :* Alzheimer's Association Alzheimer's Impact Movement, "Fact Sheet: Alzheimer's Disease Caregivers," March 2019, https://act.alz.org/site/DocServer/caregivers_fact_sheet.pdf?docID=3022.

83 *This shift cemented hospitals, in Ariès's words . . . :* Ariès, *Hour of Our Death,* 584.

83 *In 1955, the English anthropologist Geoffrey Gorer:* Geoffrey Gorer, "The Pornography of Death," *Encounter* (1955): 50–51.

84 *Today Americans are more comfortable . . . :* J. Donald Schumacher, prepared statement for "Health Care Provided to Non-Ambulatory Persons," Hearing of the Committee on Health, Education, Labor, and Pensions, US Senate, S. Hrg. 109-80, April 6, 2005, https://www.govinfo.gov/content/pkg/CHRG-109shrg20539/html/CHRG-109shrg20539.htm.

Chapter 5: Fear

94 *"Daily, round about eleven . . .":* Albert Camus, "The Plague," *The Plague, The Fall, Exile and the Kingdom, and Selected Essays,* trans. S. Gilbert (New York: Knopf, 2004), 108.

250 *Notes*

96 *In her 1978 book* Illness as Metaphor . . . : Susan Sontag, *Illness as Metaphor* (New York: Farrar, Straus and Giroux, 1977), 65–66.

96 *"in her eyes, mortality seemed as unjust as murder":* David Rieff, "Why I Had to Lie to My Dying Mother," *Guardian*, May 18, 2008, https:// www.theguardian.com/books/2008/may/18/society.

99 *"She who feared isolation . . .":* David Rieff, *Swimming in a Sea of Death: A Son's Memoir* (New York: Simon & Schuster, 2008), 151.

100 *Oregon provides us with more than . . . :* Oregon Health Authority, Public Health Division, Center for Health Statistics, "Oregon Death with Dignity Act: 2018 Data Summary," February 15, 2019, https:// www.oregon.gov/oha/PH/PROVIDERPARTNERRESOURCES /EVALUATIONRESEARCH/DEATHWITHDIGNITYACT /Documents/year21.pdf.

105 *says that pain "islands you":* Christian Wiman, "Mortify Our Wolves," *American Scholar*, Autumn 2012, https://theamericanscholar.org /mortify-our-wolves.

105 *"Let me tell you . . .":* Wiman, "Mortify Our Wolves."

105 *"one of the most uncompromising and troubling . . .":* Susan Sontag, "Simone Weil," *New York Review of Books*, February 1, 1963, http:// www.nybooks.com/articles/1963/02/01/simone-weil.

106 *"Affliction is anonymous . . .":* Simone Weil, *Waiting for God*, trans. Emma Craufurd (New York: Putnam, 1951), 125.

109 *"What accounts for the extraordinary appeal . . .":* Susan Sontag, "The Ideal Husband," *New York Review of Books*, September 26, 1963, http:// www.nybooks.com/articles/1963/09/26/the-ideal-husband.

109 *"Finally I asked . . .":* Christian Wiman, "Dying into Life," *Commonweal*, April 23, 2012, https://www.commonwealmagazine.org/dying-life.

110 *"How desperately we, the living . . .":* Wiman, "Dying into Life."

Chapter 6: Body

113 *In July 1518, a different sort . . . :* For this account of the dancing plague, I am especially indebted to John Waller, *The Dancing Plague: The Strange, True Story of an Extraordinary Illness* (Naperville, IL: Sourcebooks, 2009). I am also grateful for information from these works: Patricia Bauer, "Dancing Plague of 1518," *Encyclopedia Britannica*, May 18, 2017, https://www.britannica.com/event/dancing -plague-of-1518; Marissa Fessenden, "A Strange Case of Dancing Mania Struck Germany Six Centuries Ago Today," *Smithsonian*, June 24, 2016,

https://www.smithsonianmag.com/smart-news/strange-case-dancing
-mania-struck-germany-six-centuries-ago-today-180959549; J. F. C.
Hecker, *The Black Death and the Dancing Mania*, trans. Benjamin Guy
Babington, 1832 (CreateSpace, 2015); Neil Harding McAlister, "The
Dancing Pilgrims at Muelebeek," *Journal of the History of Medicine and
Allied Sciences* 32 (1977): 315–19.

117 *On August 16, 1951, a large number . . . :* Gabbai, Lisbonne, and
Pourquier, "Ergot Poisoning at Pont St. Esprit," *British Medical Journal*
2/4732 (September 15, 1951): 650–51. See also Jonathan N. Leonard,
"It Blew Their Minds," *New York Times,* September 8, 1968.

118 *"The delirium seemed to be systematized . . .":* Gabbai, Lisbonne, and
Pourquier, "Ergot Poisoning at Pont St. Esprit."

118 *"A worker tried to drown himself . . .":* In this section, I am indebted to
Mary Blume, "France's Unsolved Mystery of the Poisoned Bread," *New
York Times,* July 24, 2008, https://www.nytimes.com/2008/07/24/arts
/24iht-blume.1.14718462.html.

119 *Isenheim Altarpiece painted by Matthias Grünewald . . . :* For more
information about the altarpiece, see https://www.musee-unterlinden
.com/en/oeuvres/the-isenheim-altarpiece.

120 *The American novelist Francine Prose . . . :* Francine Prose, "How I
Found Life-Altering Art in Alsace," *New York Times,* July 6, 2016,
https://www.nytimes.com/2016/07/10/travel/alsace-francine
-prose.html.

120 *The Austrian-born Jewish philosopher Martin Buber . . . :* The details on
Martin Buber and Henri Matisse come from the Unterlinden Museum's
self-published book *The Isenheim Altarpiece: The Masterpiece of the
Musée Unterlinden.*

121 *"There, in the old Unterlinden convent . . .":* Joris-Karl Huysmans, "The
Grünewalds in the Colmar Museum," in *Trois Primitifs,* trans. Robert
Baldick (Oxford: Phaidon, 1958).

123 *Borrowing from Abraham Heschel . . . :* Jürgen Moltmann, *The Crucified
God: The Cross of Christ as the Foundation and Criticism of Christian
Theology* (Minneapolis: Fortress, 1993), 267–90.

125 *"Whatever it may be, one thing is certain . . .":* Huysmans, "The
Grünewalds."

127 *Instead, he tells Martha . . . :* John 11:24–25 (NRSV).

128 *"Imagine yourself in hospital with chest pains . . .":* John Hare, "My God,
My God, Why Have You Forsaken Me?" Palm Sunday sermon text,
St. John's Episcopal Church, New Haven, CT, 2018.

Chapter 7: Spirit

138 *"Americans May Be Getting Less Religious . . .":* David Masci and Michael
     Lipka, "Americans May Be Getting Less Religious, but Feelings of
     Spirituality Are on the Rise," *Pew Research Center*, January 21, 2016,
     http://www.pewresearch.org/fact-tank/2016/01/21/americans
     -spirituality.

138 *The free-spirited, individualistic baby boomers . . . :* Richard N. Ostling,
     "The Church Search," *Time*, April 5, 1993, 44.

139 *Gen Xers are trying to make sense of the world . . . :* Ralph Ryback, "From
     Baby Boomers to Generation Z: The Generational Gaps and Their
     Roles in Society," *Psychology Today*, February 22, 2016, https://www
     .psychologytoday.com/us/blog/the-truisms-wellness/201602/baby
     -boomers-generation-z.

139 *Finally, we have the Millennials—the "least religious generation":* Beth
     Downing Chee, "The Least Religious Generation," *SDSU NewsCenter*,
     May 27, 2015, http://newscenter.sdsu.edu/sdsu_newscenter/news
     _story.aspx?sid=75623.

139 *Millennials are less likely to be religious . . . :* Jean M. Twenge et al.,
     "Generational and Time Period Differences in American Adolescents'
     Religious Orientation, 1966–2014," *PLoS ONE* 10/5 (May 11, 2015):
     e0121454, doi:10.1371/journal.pone.0121454.

139 *Wright describes three main beliefs . . . :* N. T. Wright, *Surprised by Hope:
     Rethinking Heaven, the Resurrection, and the Mission of the Church* (San
     Francisco: HarperOne, 2008), 9–12.

140 *"There is no soul . . .":* Shelly Kagan, *Death*, Open Yale Courses Series
     (New Haven, CT: Yale Univ. Press, 2012), 363.

142 *Take the Canadian social worker . . . :* Catherine Porter, "At His Own
     Wake, Celebrating Life and the Gift of Death," *New York Times*,
     May 25, 2017, https://www.nytimes.com/2017/05/25/world/canada
     /euthanasia-bill-john-shields-death.html.

142 *Religious studies professor Robert Fuller . . . :* Robert C. Fuller, *Spiritual,
     but Not Religious: Understanding Unchurched America* (New York:
     Oxford Univ. Press, 2001), 12.

143 *Fuller is quick to note that SBNR individuals . . . :* Fuller, *Spiritual, but
     Not Religious*, 8.

144 *However, she goes on to admit . . . :* Lillian Daniel, *When "Spiritual but
     Not Religious" Is Not Enough: Seeing God in Surprising Places, Even the
     Church* (New York: Jericho, 2013), 12.

144 *Yet she argues that a religious . . . :* Daniel, *When "Spiritual but Not Religious" Is Not Enough*, 13.

145 *Jon Levenson, Harvard professor of Jewish studies . . . :* Jon D. Levenson, *Resurrection and the Restoration of Israel: The Ultimate Victory of the God of Life* (New Haven, CT: Yale Univ. Press, 2006), ix.

146 *But most first-century Jews believed . . . :* In this section also I am indebted to Wright, *Surprised by Hope*, 37.

146 *No Jewish person at the time . . . :* Wright, *Surprised by Hope*, 34.

146 *"a weight-bearing beam . . .":* Levenson, *Resurrection and the Restoration*, x.

146 *"Without the restoration of the people Israel . . .":* Levenson, *Resurrection and the Restoration*, x.

146 *This uprooted deep cultural assumptions . . . :* Wright, *Surprised by Hope*, 37

146 *It went from being a vague notion . . . :* Wright, *Surprised by Hope*, 42–47.

148 *"by excluding the resurrection of the dead . . .":* Levenson, *Resurrection and the Restoration*, 3.

148 *Levenson and coauthor Kevin Madigan argue . . . :* Kevin J. Madigan and Jon Douglas Levenson, *Resurrection: The Power of God for Christians and Jews* (New Haven, CT: Yale Univ. Press, 2009), 115.

151 *Wiman characterizes himself in his earlier years . . . :* Christian Wiman, "I Will Love You in the Summertime," *American Scholar*, February 29, 2016, https://theamericanscholar.org/i-will-love-you-in-the-summertime /#.WxnSelLMxE4.

151 *"One doesn't follow God in hope of happiness . . .":* Wiman, "I Will Love You."

Chapter 8: Ritual

154 *"social architecture that marks . . .":* David Brooks, "There Should Be More Rituals!" *New York Times*, April 22, 2019, https://www.nytimes .com/2019/04/22/opinion/rituals-meaning.html.

158 *Cremation rates vary widely around the world:* The Cremation Society in the UK collects international data on cremation rates. See https://www .cremation.org.uk for more information.

158 *At the time of her interview with the* Guardian *. . . :* Jenn Park-Mustacchio, "I've Been an Embalmer for 14 Years and See My Share of Bodies. Any Questions?" *Guardian*, October 24, 2013, https:// www.theguardian.com/commentisfree/2013/oct/24/embalmer-for -14-years-ask-me-anything.

159 *It is especially satisfying, she says . . . :* Park-Mustacchio, "I've Been an Embalmer."

160 *The journalist Jessica Mitford . . . :* Jessica Mitford, *The American Way of Death Revisited* (New York: Vintage, 1998), 43.

161 Tahara *is the ritual of cleansing . . . :* See Catherine Madsen, "Love Songs to the Dead: The Liturgical Voice as Mentor and Reminder," *Cross Currents* 48/4 (Winter 1998–99): 458–59.

163 *"no Freud, no television . . .":* Madsen, "Love Songs to the Dead."

164 *"If the lines had not been in the ritual . . .":* Madsen, "Love Songs to the Dead."

164 *The acclaimed writer Anita Diamant . . . :* Mayyim Hayyim; see https://www.mayyimhayyim.org.

164 *On the opposite coast, Rabbi Avivah Erlick . . . :* For Sacred Waters, see https://www.rabbiavivah.com/sacred-waters-2.

166 *For many people, the idea of funeral as theater . . . :* Stella Adler, *The Art of Acting* (New York: Applause, 2000), 29.

166 *The theater, she says, is where people see . . . :* Adler, *Art of Acting*, 30.

166 *In his book on funerals Thomas Long . . . :* This section is taken from: Thomas G. Long, *Accompany Them with Singing—The Christian Funeral* (Louisville, KY: Westminster John Knox, 2013): 122–23.

167 *"The ideas of the great playwrights . . .":* Adler, *Art of Acting*, 65.

168 *"This saint, though deceased . . .":* Long, *Accompany Them with Singing*, 154.

170 *And to do so requires . . . :* Long, *Accompany Them with Singing*, 158–59.

175 *"Throughout each afternoon and evening . . .":* Personal communication with Rabbi Eliana Falk, January 2, 2018.

176 *"We are commanded not to engage . . .":* Jonathan Sacks, "The Limits of Grief (Re'eh 5777)," August 14, 2017, http://rabbisacks.org/limits-grief-reeh-5777.

Chapter 9: Life

180 *even if some scientists explain it as . . . :* For more on this, see Carol Zaleski, *The Life of the World to Come: Near-Death Experience and Christian Hope*, Albert Cardinal Meyer Lectures (Oxford: Oxford Univ. Press, 1996).

184 *the assessment developed by the geriatrician Linda Fried . . . :* Linda P. Fried et al., "Frailty in Older Adults: Evidence for a Phenotype," *Journal of Gerontology: Medical Sciences* 56/3 (March 2001): M146–56.

185 *Another study found that among older cancer patients . . . :* C. Handforth et al., "The Prevalence and Outcomes of Frailty in Older

Cancer Patients: A Systematic Review," *Annals of Oncology* 26/6 (June 2015): 1091–101.

186 *A group of Yale physicians found . . . :* John M. Thomas, Leo M. Cooney Jr., and Terri R. Fried, "Systematic Review: Health-related Characteristics of Elderly Hospitalized Patients and Nursing Home Residents Associated with Short-term Mortality," *Journal of the American Geriatrics Society* 61/6 (June 2013): 902–11.

189 *"Of all the professions, medicine is . . .":* Sherwin Nuland, *How We Die* (New York: Knopf, 1994), 258.

191 *Nuland's ninety-two-year-old patient . . . :* Nuland, *How We Die*, 250–53.

192 *a famous study published by a group of doctors . . . :* Jennifer S. Temel et al., "Early Palliative Care for Patients with Metastatic Non-Small-Cell Lung Cancer," *New England Journal of Medicine* 363/8 (2010): 733–42.

195 *But in the real world, CPR works far less often . . . :* J. Portanova et al., "It Isn't Like This on TV: Revisiting CPR Survival Rates Depicted on Popular TV Shows," *Resuscitation* 96 (2015): 148–50.

196 *A group of Boston researchers looked at . . . :* A. El-Jawahri et al., "A Randomized Controlled Trial of a CPR and Intubation Video Decision Support Tool for Hospitalized Patients," *Journal of General Internal Medicine* 30/8 (2015): 1071–80.

200 *Studies have shown that having purpose in life . . . :* Paula Span, "Living on Purpose," *New York Times,* June 3, 2014, https://newoldage.blogs .nytimes.com/2014/06/03/living-on-purpose.

200 *"Manny was older and frailer . . .":* Span, "Living on Purpose."

201 *Forty percent of Americans say that . . . :* "Where Americans Find Meaning in Life," *Pew Research Center,* November 20, 2018, http:// www.pewforum.org/2018/11/20/where-americans-find-meaning-in -life; Patrick Van Kessel and Adam Hughes, "Americans Who Find Meaning in These Four Areas Have Higher Life Satisfaction," *Pew Research Center,* November 20, 2018, http://www.pewresearch.org /fact-tank/2018/11/20/americans-who-find-meaning-in-these-four -areas-have-higher-life-satisfaction.

202 *The Pew Research Center recently attempted . . . :* "Where Americans Find Meaning in Life."

207 *The mid-twentieth-century chaplain . . . :* Peter Marshall, *John Doe, Disciple* (New York: McGraw Hill, 1963).

212 *"When a group of people sing together . . .":* Andy Fuller, "Coda," Office of Public Affairs and Communications, University of Notre Dame, https://www.nd.edu/stories/coda.

213 *One of the earliest literary records of last words . . . :* See Gen. 49–50 (NRSV).
214 *"Dying was not merely . . .":* For this section on Methodist biographies I am indebted to Shai J. Lavi, *The Modern Art of Dying: A History of Euthanasia in the United States* (Princeton, NJ: Princeton Univ. Press, 2005), 27.
215 *Leonardo da Vinci's last words . . . :* Giorgio Vasari, *The Life of Leonardo da Vinci*, trans. Herbert P. Horne (New York: Longmans Green, 1903), 44.
215 *Thomas Edison, long considered . . . :* Neil Baldwin, *Edison: Inventing the Century* (Chicago: Univ. of Chicago Press, 2001), 407.
215 *"Oh wow. Oh wow. Oh wow.":* Mona Simpson, "A Sister's Eulogy for Steve Jobs," *New York Times*, October 30, 2011, https://www.nytimes.com/2011/10/30/opinion/mona-simpsons-eulogy-for-steve-jobs.html.

L. S. Dugdale, MD, MAR, is associate professor of medicine and director of the Center for Clinical Medical Ethics at Columbia University. Prior to her 2019 move to Columbia, she was associate director of the Program for Biomedical Ethics and founding codirector of the Program for Medicine, Spirituality, and Religion at Yale School of Medicine. She is an internal medicine primary care doctor and medical ethicist. Her first book, *Dying in the Twenty-First Century* (MIT Press, 2015), provides the theoretical grounding for this current book. She lives with her husband and daughters in New York City.

Michael W. Dugger is an artist who works in multiple media. He is a graduate of Interlochen Arts Academy and Western Michigan University. He lives in York, Pennsylvania. Michael is also a firefighter and medic; from this context he is familiar with the mechanics and apparatus of death. See more of his work at mwdugger.com.